Yoga Mama Yoga Baby

AUDIO PROGRAM BY MARGO SHAPIRO BACHMAN

*Yoga Mama, Yoga Baby: Complete Practices
for Every Stage of Pregnancy and Birth*

MARGO SHAPIRO BACHMAN

Yoga Mama Yoga Baby

AYURVEDA AND YOGA FOR A HEALTHY PREGNANCY AND BIRTH

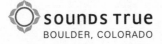

sounds true
BOULDER, COLORADO

Sounds True, Inc.
Boulder, CO 80306

This work is solely for personal growth and education. It should not be treated as a substitute for professional assistance or medical advice. Any attempt to diagnose or treat an illness should be done under the direction of a health-care professional. The application of protocols and information in this book is the choice of each reader, who assumes full responsibility for his or her understandings, interpretations, and results. Should the reader have any questions concerning the appropriateness of any procedure or preparation mentioned, the author and publisher strongly suggest consulting a professional healthcare advisor. The author and publisher assume no responsibility for the actions or choices of any reader.

Cover and book design by Rachael Murray
Cover photo © vlavetal, shutterstock.com

Printed in the United States of America

The lists "Dirty Dozen" and "Clean Fifteen" on page 246 are Copyright © Environmental Working Group, ewg.org. Reprinted with permission.

Library of Congress Cataloging-in-Publication Data
Bachman, Margo Shapiro.
  Yoga mama, yoga baby : ayurveda and yoga for a healthy pregnancy and birth / Margo Shapiro
    Bachman, MA.
      pages cm
  Includes bibliographical references and index.
  ISBN 978-1-60407-985-2
  1. Exercise for pregnant women. 2. Active childbirth. 3. Hatha yoga. 4. Medicine, Ayurvedic. I.
    Title.
  RG558.7.B33 2013
  618.2'44--dc23
                                                2013015344

Ebook ISBN 978-1-62203-068-2

10 9 8 7 6 5 4

This book is dedicated to all women.
May your pregnancies be joyful, peaceful, and radiantly healthy.

Contents

CONTENTS

Every woman has an inner awareness of what it is like to be a mother. In the true sense, every woman is a divine mother, whether she has a child or not; it does not matter. The essence of Mother is present in every woman as sharing, caring, loving, and forgiving. In *Yoga Mama, Yoga Baby* Margo Bachman beautifully elaborates the basic principles of Ayurveda—the science of life—and combines it with the complete practice of yoga. Using the fundamental principles of these two disciplines, the prospective mother is led through exercises, practices, and inner exploration to awaken inner bliss, joy, and fulfillment as she advances through her pregnancy.

Ayurveda and yoga are concurrent and inherent. They are sister disciplines that bring health and happiness, helping one to achieve the four pillars of life: *dharma* (duty), *artha* (wealth), *kama* (desire), and *moksha* (enlightenment).

Both Ayurveda and yoga have eight limbs, or branches, of disciplines. Ayurveda has eight branches of internal medicine: medicine; surgery; ear, nose, and throat; gynecology; obstetrics; pediatrics; geriatrics; and psychospiritual healing. Yoga's eight branches, known as *ashtanga* yoga, are *yama* (social ethics), *niyama* (personal self-care), *asana* (physical postures), *pranayama* (breath regulation), *pratyahara* (withdrawal of the senses), *dharana* (concentration), *dhyana* (meditation), and *samadhi* (complete absorption into universal consciousness). These eight limbs are skillfully applied in this book.

The View of Ayurveda

Ayurveda is an ancient Vedic system of healing based upon six systems of philosophy, out of which Ayurveda has completely accepted *Sankhya's* philosophy. According to this system, *purusha*—pure, choiceless, passive awareness—and *prakruti*—primordial matter—combine to make up the first evolution of creation into supreme intelligence, which is called *mahat*. Mahat has no identity or center. It is cosmic intelligence that permeates all of creation. Mahat further manifests as *ahamkar,* the awareness of one's own existence, the sense of "I am," of having an identity or a center.

Whenever you look at a bowl, whether it is gold, silver, or wood, you might see just the substance of the bowl—the gold, silver, or wood. But in Ayurveda, we look at the form. Form is spiritual and substance is material. We don't look at the material aspect of the substance but deeply penetrate into the spiritual existence of it. Ayurveda embraces every aspect of experienced reality—this feeling of "I am" is expressed in three qualities that encompass all of creation: the observer, the observation, and the thing to be observed. This whole universe is expressed from the formless into form, from the nameless into name. We have a name for everything: the cloud, the mountain, the bird, the tree, the flower. Everything has a unique form and everything has a name. According to this philosophy of creation, the journey of consciousness into matter happens through *namarupa,* through the name and the form.

This book teaches these ancient philosophies with clinical and practical levels of application. Margo gives us Ayurveda, the science of life, with its profound knowledge of the physical body. She presents the important facts about the prakruti, doshas, and elements. Prakruti is our unique genetic code, which is the permutation and combination of both a qualitative and quantitative mixture of the three doshas: *vata, pitta, kapha.*

Our prakruti is our individual constitution and it expresses as a combination of the three doshas—a person can be mono-doshic, dual-doshic, or triple-doshic. This is the qualitative expression. The subtle body expresses the vital essence of the doshas as *prana, tejas,* and *ojas.* These are the pure essences of the doshas: prana is the pure essence of vata dosha, tejas is of pitta dosha, and ojas is of kapha dosha. They function at a deep, cellular level. These govern the functional activity of the body, mind, and consciousness.

However, the structural aspects of the body, mind, and consciousness are governed by the five elements: ether, air, fire, water, and earth. They are present in the universe (macrocosm) as well as in the structure in every cell, as the functional units of the human body (microcosm). These spaces include the cranial space, thoracic space, and abdominal and pelvic space. Pelvic space is related to air, supra pelvic space to water, abdominal space—including the stomach and its digestive enzymes—to fire, thoracic space to air, and space in the brain is related to ether. Each of the three doshas results from a unique permutation and combination of the five elements. All five elements are present in each dosha, but vata is primarily a combination of ether and air, pitta is of fire and water, and kapha is made up of water and earth. In her book, Margo Bachman has expertly expressed this picture of the elements and the doshas, as well as prana, tejas, ojas, and sattva, rajas, tamas.

Well-Being through Yoga

In this book, the focal point of yoga practice is focused upon the individual's unique constitution with this understanding of the three Ayurvedic doshas. Ultimately, through yogic discipline, we have to bring these wandering doshas back to their "homes" of vata in the pelvic cavity, pitta in the abdominal cavity, and kapha in the thoracic cavity. When we balance the doshas *in situ,* then everything from the conception of the child to pre- and post-natal care becomes easy.

The complete practice of yoga would require all eight limbs of this discipline. But to the pregnant mother, Margo teaches aspects of yoga that are safe for mother and baby, including practical directions for a complete yoga practice during the prenatal period that encompass yoga postures, breathing techniques, and meditation. She has chosen yoga practices that bring coordination, synchronization, tone, and power of the muscles— both in prenatal yoga postures and breathing techniques called *pranayama.*

Another profound practice of great benefit is pranayama, or yogic deep-breathing exercises. Prana is the vital breath and vital air; it is life. By doing pranayama, one can bring rhythm into the breath. Prana and *manas* (mind) are intimately connected. The mind governs prana and prana governs the mind—they are the two sides of the same coin. By doing pranayama, we bring harmony to our thinking, feeling, and emotions. Pranayama strengthens prana, building ojas and tejas. Pranayama brings harmony at the cellular level to ojas, tejas, and prana, at the doshic level to vata, pitta, and kapha, and at the physiological level to the *dhatus* (tissues) and *malas* (wastes).

Margo Bachman has offered specific pranayamas for specific conditions. The practices of pranayama she recommends help to bring relaxation, calmness, and tranquility to the pregnant mother so that she develops courage and has confidence at the time of labor. In this way, the important spiritual and yogic discipline of pranayama has a great therapeutic value. When a woman practices pranayama before pregnancy, during pregnancy, and during delivery, she enables the passage (birth canal), passenger (the child), and pressure (uterine contractions) to work together harmoniously to make the journey safe.

A Harmonious and Balanced Pregnancy

With this book, the expectant mother has specific guidelines for each trimester regarding diet and lifestyle measures that will help to build ojas. Another aspect of pregnancy that Margo teaches is exploring and deepening intimacy with your partner, which is beneficial. Some of the breathing practices balance one's male and female energy and help to unfold intimacy and balance in relationship.

There is deep connection between mind and breath. Breathing is the physiological part of the respiration, while thinking is the psychological part of breathing. Thinking and breathing are intimately connected. To harness this, Margo has offered a very deep meditation called *So Hum*. So Hum is very powerful; it is a natural mantra that is singing in the breath of every individual. During the act of inhalation, the sound of "so" goes in, which is the Shiva energy—the divine consciousness. During the act of exhalation, the sound of "hum" goes out. "Hum" is the energy of the ego—the individual consciousness.

In So Hum breathing, there is a silent gap between So and Hum if you pause after the inhalation of So, and before the exhalation of Hum. Similarly, when Hum comes out and before it becomes the So of inhalation, there is also a silent gap. There are two gaps: one behind the belly button (So) and one outside the body (Hum). By pausing, for a split second you exist without breath, you exist without time, and you exist without mind. Mind is the movement of breath, and in that gap, there is no time because movement of breath is time. Resting in this gap can help the mother to bear the pain of uterine contractions during delivery. This is a practical application of So Hum meditation before delivery and during labor pain.

Yoga Mama, Yoga Baby is a practical guide for both mom and baby to bring harmony among body, mind, and consciousness. Yogic discipline, Ayurvedic diet and lifestyle guidelines, and simple domestic herbal plans provide effective methods for a healthy, happy pregnancy and healthy, happy child. Plan positively and create a divine invitation to a divine soul through the practical application of this book.

Vasant Lad, BAMS, MASc
Founder of The Ayurvedic Institute
Albuquerque, November 2013

INTRODUCTION

I consider motherhood as one of my *dharmas* in this lifetime. *Dharma* is a Sanskrit word that means a duty, responsibility, or purpose to our society, our families, and ourselves. Each of us has many dharmas, or roles, in life that support us if we act to support them. Like many women, I'd always had an inherent desire to experience pregnancy, birth, motherhood, and family life. When I was younger, motherhood always seemed distant, but as the third decade of my life approached, it beckoned. My husband and I had found each other and married, and I felt ready to embark on this new journey. As an alternative healthcare provider and longtime yoga practitioner, I wanted my pregnancy journey to be guided by the wisdom of yoga and Ayurveda.

After spending over a decade immersed in the study of Western herbal medicine, I revisited my longtime interest in Ayurveda, which integrated well with herbalism and improved my understanding of health and wellness. This interest led me to spend years in private and small-group studies with some of the pioneers in the field of Ayurveda today, including Dr. Vasant Lad, Maya Tiwari, and Dr. David Frawley. These extraordinary teachers shaped my education, inspired my clinical practice, and helped me to understand myself. Each one contributed something uniquely different and compelling to my Ayurvedic education. I was and continue to be blessed by my mentorship with Dr. Frawley, a leading expert on Ayurveda and other Indian sciences, who took me under his wing and carefully guided my work on many levels.

Yoga, Ayurveda's sister science, has been an integral part of my life for almost fifteen years, through studying, practicing, and teaching in a variety of contexts with different populations. My interest in yoga brought me to the Krishnamacharya Yoga Mandiram, one of the leading educational institutions for yoga therapy in India, and Sonia Nelson (a senior teacher in the lineage of T. K. V. Desikachar and T. Krishnamacharya) continues to mentor and support me today.

With the tools and insights of herbal medicine, yoga, and Ayurveda, I felt ready to prepare my body for conception and pregnancy. I took herbs renowned for nourishing and toning the female reproductive system and building the tissues and blood, including shatavari, vidari, raspberry leaf, and nettles. I changed my daily yoga practices to focus on opening my hips and pelvis, preparing my body for an easier pregnancy and birth, and performed a short round of *panchakarma* (Ayurvedic deep detoxification and rejuvenation therapy), which is often done to prepare for conception. My husband and I conceived our daughter on our first try, and we were ecstatic.

My first pregnancy was truly a joyous experience. By keeping my diet, herbal support, and lifestyle in harmony with my Ayurvedic constitution (the individual combination of physical, mental, and emotional characteristics), I rarely felt sick or fatigued. My mind was focused on my baby's health and my own. When imbalances did arise, I relied on simple Ayurvedic remedies and the tools of yoga, which worked extremely well. I made the pregnancy my highest priority and did whatever I could to honor the sacred process of gestation.

Because I'd had a healthy and easy pregnancy, I presumed that birth would be a seamless extension of it and that the baby would pop out in a birthing tub in our bedroom. But it did not play out the way I had envisioned. My water broke with no contractions. To help my labor along, I tried one natural method after another, from castor oil and herbs to acupuncture to dancing and prayers. Nothing kicked my labor into full gear. After twenty-four hours and only very mild contractions, my labor was still not progressing, and I started showing meconium, which can indicate fetal distress. Our midwife informed us that I needed to be transported to the hospital and labor would need to be induced.

Since I had not slept in twenty-four hours, when I received my first dose of Pitocin, I had no reserves to tolerate the artificial hormone. I tried to keep up with the rapidly intensifying contractions, but the force was so great that my body could not relax to dilate further. My eyes welled up with tears as I saw myself confined to a hospital bed with three intravenous needles in my arm and a belt around my stomach. As an earthy, natural person my whole life, I'd wanted to experience the sensations of natural contractions and squatting to push my child out in a comforting setting. Being in the sterile hospital, with all the accouterments of modern medicine, was not part of my vision! Eventually, I received an epidural and went to sleep.

A few hours later, my body was ready. In retrospect, I am thankful for the resources available, because they helped me to progress and successfully birth my daughter, Sierra. We were both healthy, and that was what mattered. This birth experience was my first exposure to the uncertainty of motherhood and a true experience of surrendering to what was out of my control. I now see that I had neglected to practice the yoga principles of *tapas, svadhyaya,* and *ishvara pranidhana,* which roughly translate to the practices of first making an effort to do something, then observing yourself in action, and finally adopting an attitude of not being attached to the fruits of your actions and accepting whatever happens. I was holding on too tightly to the end result I'd envisioned, and that attachment created an incredible struggle for me. If I would have remembered these important principles, I may have had a completely different, more positive experience.

My husband, daughter, and I spent our first year together bonding while I learned a great deal about myself and daughter, along with the ins and outs of parenthood. A few years later, when my husband and I decided we wanted another child, once again, with preparation and intention, we conceived quickly.

I felt great until one night in the sixth week, when I had a dream that the baby was not alive. I woke up disoriented and confused. The dream felt very real. I tried to ignore the thoughts that the baby was not alive, but my intuition told me that something was not right. At ten weeks, I went for an ultrasound and sadly discovered there was no fetal heartbeat. The fetus had stopped growing around six weeks of gestation, just when I had the dream.

I continually asked myself how and why this miscarriage could have happened. My husband and I were both very healthy. I knew there was no direct explanation, but I felt very heavyhearted and disappointed. The experience shed light on how dreams are one of the ways our intuition communicates with us. I tapped into yoga and Ayurveda to help with my grieving process and trauma recovery by adopting a positive attitude based on yogic principles, using simple *pranayama* practices to lift and transform sadness, and using herbs for emotional and hormonal balance and clearing stagnation after the miscarriage. Eventually, I came to terms with the loss.

After several months of recovering from the physical and emotional trauma of that experience, my husband and I wanted to conceive again. This time it did not happen as easily. Was there scar tissue from the miscarriage? Had my hormones reset properly? I questioned whether or not I was actually ovulating. Tired after months of regularly scheduled lovemaking during my fertile period, we decided to let go of the effort and move on with other aspects of our lives. I became pregnant the next month.

However, this pregnancy was quite different from the previous two. The classic nausea and vomiting in the first trimester were my new world. Mine did not start in the morning, but began after lunch and lasted until I went to bed at night. Sometimes I would wake up woozy in the middle of the night. I could no longer stomach the beautiful, healthy meals that had been my staple during my first pregnancy. I prepared them for my daughter and husband, but became nauseated by the smell of the food. I settled on bagels and cream cheese.

This experience helped me realize that women in sound health do not always feel well when they're pregnant. I relied heavily on simple Ayurvedic remedies and the tools of yoga to feel stronger and more balanced. I also learned that our attitude toward the imbalances and discomfort is just as important as the tools we use to address them. Our ability to adapt to the situation at hand is crucial.

After the first trimester, the nausea subsided, and the rest of the pregnancy was smooth. However, I knew I did not want to repeat the same scenario of my first birth. I felt that it was my right as a woman to experience natural childbirth, and I became determined to do all I could (within my means) to achieve this. I wanted to feel the pulse of every contraction and the extraordinary magic of giving birth with minimal to no intervention.

I had two insights that I didn't have during my first birth: (1) the knowledge to keep my endurance strong with yoga and other forms of exercise through the entire pregnancy and (2) labor support in the form of a doula. Both of these served me well, and my son, Mateo, popped out easily after five hours of intense and exhilarating natural labor.

Both of my birthing experiences taught me invaluable lessons, especially in how to surrender and to empower myself. In my first birth, I had to yield to the river of life. It was all I could do to bring my baby into my arms. In my second birth, I tapped into a deep reserve of inner strength that I honestly did not know I had within me. These experiences gave me more strength and ability to face life than anything had given me before. Both rites of passage made me a different woman than I was before each child.

How This Book Was Conceived

After the birth of my first child, I decided to devote my yoga and Ayurveda practice to women and children's health. I dove deeply into the classical texts of Ayurveda and yoga to see what wisdom could be gleaned from these ancient sciences. I found myself continually asking, "How can I bridge these primordial teachings into useful, meaningful, and practical tools for modern women and families?" I looked for a book on yoga and Ayurveda for pregnancy and birth, but was surprised to find a void in this area of literature. Of all the pregnancy books on the market today, very few provide practical and sensible support from Ayurveda and yoga *together* to help women experience joyful and healthy pregnancies. I realized that I needed to write the book I was searching for.

The result, which you hold in your hands, blends my direct studies with renowned teachers of Ayurveda and yoga, research of classical texts from India, clinical experience working with pregnant clients, and personal experiences during my pregnancies. The basic principle of Ayurveda is that the body can and will heal itself, when it is given the right effort, tools, and guidance. In my years of counseling women in the childbearing stage of life, and addressing the myriad potential accompanying health challenges, I have seen time and time again how the natural wisdom of Ayurveda and yoga work effectively to restore health and bring balance to countless areas of life.

How Yoga and Ayurveda Can Guide Your Pregnancy

Yoga and Ayurveda are sister sciences that have been connected for thousands of years. Steeped in the same philosophy, they provide important, complementary tools and practices for creating a healthy body, a balanced mind, and higher consciousness. They promote a healthy, natural lifestyle through diet, herbs, physical postures, and breathing techniques. They also include prayers, chants, and meditation, and promote certain ethical values, such as truthfulness, nonviolence, and humility. But neither requires you to follow certain deities, dogmas, or religions.

The holistic diet and lifestyle recommendations of yoga and Ayurveda begin with understanding your unique constitution and how to live in harmony with it. *Self-knowledge and self-care are central principles of Ayurveda and are key to real, deep, and lasting healing and health.* Many times, imbalances arise as a result of diet and lifestyle choices that aren't appropriate for our unique nature. By understanding your constitution, you can pay attention to your needs and make choices that support your health and well-being.

In pregnancy specifically, yoga and Ayurveda can help you improve the quality of your life, enjoy the process of gestation, and raise your consciousness, as well as achieve optimum health for yourself and your growing baby.

On a practical level, yoga and Ayurveda, as forms of natural medicine, provide specific tools for helping with the challenges that can arise during pregnancy. I have met countless women who really dislike being pregnant. They feel uncomfortable, sick, or exhausted, or suffer from a host of conditions for anywhere from a few weeks to their entire pregnancy. Some women feel hindered and don't like to feel slowed down. Others feel awkward in their pregnant bodies and don't enjoy their fullness or how their body is morphing to accommodate their growing baby. And a number of women feel that their hormones have hijacked their bodies and emotions. These are all natural and genuine responses to pregnancy. Yoga and Ayurveda offer simple breath and movement techniques, gentle herbs, and basic dietary suggestions to help you ride these changing tides.

On a more profound level, Ayurveda suggests that the prenatal environment influences your baby's *prakruti*, or constitution. Both in the womb and out, a child's consciousness, health, and happiness are shaped by its parents' activities, diet, lifestyle, and mental states. Ayurveda and yoga help you give your little one as much positivity as possible when she's in the womb, so she may come into this world as strong and healthy as can be. In addition, yoga helps you to become more present with yourself, moment by moment, day after day—an invaluable skill that can serve you well during birth and motherhood.

Pregnancy and Birth as Rites of Passage

The principles and practices of both Ayurveda and yoga can help you honor pregnancy and birth as important rites of passage—and honor yourself as you move through them.

A rite of passage is a ritual or ceremony to honor a significant juncture in life. Rites of passage have the potential to be incredibly powerful, if we take the opportunity to make them sacred. Then they can allow us to navigate through a transition and into a new phase of life with intention, confidence, and grace.

Births, weddings, and deaths are life-changing events, and various communities and religious groups honor them with specific traditions. In the process, these traditions help link an individual to friends, family, and the larger society. However, some significant transitions in a woman's life, such as menarche, pregnancy, and menopause, are not given as much attention, especially in our modern Western culture. All of these junctures affect a woman's physical, psychological, and spiritual self, and all have the potential to connect or disconnect her from others. By acknowledging all of these significant life transitions, especially through ritual, women feel supported, honored, and prepared as they move through them.

When a woman views her pregnancy as a rite of passage, it helps her recognize that her life is changing significantly. She is moving from mother-to-be to mother, an inherent transformation in a woman's being. Honoring this transition helps a woman to truly value her experience and process of pregnancy, become empowered by it, and move through it from a place of harmony and security.

Our modern society generally views pregnancy as an individual's responsibility instead of a community's responsibility. Pregnant women often feel isolated and alone. Even though pregnancy is a woman's *own* inner journey with herself and her growing baby, comfort and support can come from her community. When pregnant women come together for something as simple as a childbirth-preparation class or a prenatal yoga class, they feel supported and more connected to the whole of life. I remember meeting some extraordinary women in those classes. We shared our secrets for itchy bellies and how we handled our nesting instincts. These classes became opportunities to connect with other women going through a similar transition and laid a foundation for relationships that continued to develop after birth.

Birth is a rite of passage in and of itself. Birthing is a complex, intense experience that can forever change a woman's existence. The actual act is a profound initiation into motherhood. Our culture today often gives baby gifts to recognize new mothers after the baby arrives, yet little attention is given to what a woman has just gone through—physically, emotionally, and spiritually—to bring the baby into the world. The rite of passage of birth is often overlooked. Instead of more baby blankets, what women need is someone to listen to them, comfort them, make them a mug of tea or a pot of soup, and rub their backs as they adjust to their new identity as mothers.

With the principles and practices of yoga and Ayurveda, you can view your pregnancy and birthing as rites of passage and navigate them with intention and insight. Hopefully, with this awareness, you can move through these transitions connected to the inner light within you and the collective strength and wisdom of all women who have made these passages before you.

Several aspects of this book can help you honor pregnancy and birth as rites of passage. The journaling exercises, for example, can help you to reflect on how your life is changing by bringing more awareness and insights to your experiences. The *asana* practices can help you to feel comfortable in your body so you can move forward with grace and confidence. The meditations assist in deeply supporting the different stages of your pregnancy with intentions. And the sound practices can help you to vocalize supportive phrases to empower yourself.

How to Use This Book

This book is a guide to help you experience radiant health and abundant joy during your pregnancy and birth. The exercises and practices are intended to spark your own self-discovery and help you to move inward during your personal journey. The book can help you access your intuition, reflect on your process, and become more present, enabling you to achieve a deeper state of wellness and encounter the powerful, wise, intuitive woman inside of yourself.

Part one, "The Basics," introduces you to the fundamentals of Ayurvedic and yogic diet and lifestyle, giving you the foundation you need to make use of the exercises, practices, and other juicy info in part two, "Your Pregnancy: A Month-by-Month Guide." Part three, "Birth and Postpartum," includes practical tips to encourage natural labor, and guidance on staying healthy and happy during the precious and tender first weeks with your baby. The appendices include suggestions for treating common pregnancy complaints with simple home remedies, delicious recipes to try, and other supplementary support.

If you are unclear or unsure about anything presented in this book, consult with your doctor, midwife, yoga teacher, Ayurvedic practitioner, or other healthcare provider. This book is not a replacement for any direct care.

You will want to purchase a notebook for the journaling exercises. Keep it accessible along with a good pen, sharpened pencil, and any other tools you will use, like colored pencils. Feel free to use the journal at other times for your thoughts, feelings, and reflections. Some women enjoy journaling after the meditation practices to further process new insights.

You may wish to stock a fresh supply of many of the herbs and spices mentioned throughout the book, so you will have what you need at your fingertips. Creating your own herbal pantry and refreshing your kitchen spice collection is fun and empowering. Many herbs and spices—such as nettles, raspberry leaf, milky oats, ginger root, cardamom pods, and cinnamon sticks—make delicious teas and additions to your food, and can be used freely throughout your pregnancy. Store herbs and spices in clean, dry, glass jars, out of direct light and away from heat.

Generally, most herbs traditionally used to support pregnancy are safe when used in moderation. Consuming normal amounts of spices in your cooking is typically considered harmless. There have been almost no reports of gentle herbs traditionally used to support pregnancy causing adverse outcomes in pregnant women, when used as directed. When negative outcomes have occurred, it has been from herbs that are *not* considered safe in pregnancy, or from products that have been contaminated with unsafe herbs, mostly from products imported from China and India. The resources section lists reputable companies that test their herbs for heavy metals, and offer organic, sustainably sourced, and high-quality products.

My Gift to You

I hope you enjoy reading this book and treasure every moment of your pregnancy. It truly is an extraordinary season in your life that deserves special attention and guidance. My greatest wish and most sincere desire is that the light of knowledge in this book will help you experience joy and excellent health in your pregnancy, so that more babies will be birthed into the world with radiant health, genuine happiness, higher consciousness, and divine love.

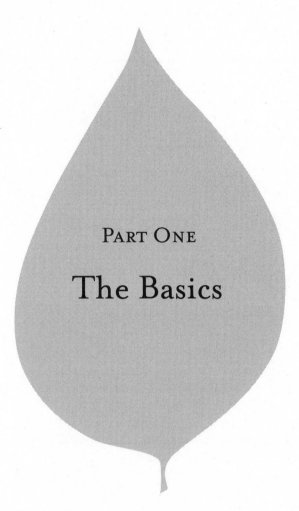

PART ONE

The Basics

Ayurveda,
the Science of Life

It is health that is real wealth and not pieces of gold and silver.
MAHATMA GANDHI

Over twenty years ago, I drove from Washington State to New Mexico to backpack in a wilderness area with a couple of girlfriends from college. We stopped by the Ayurvedic Institute in Albuquerque to see what it was all about. At the time, it was one of the few schools of Ayurveda in the US. They graciously invited us into their main class-room to hear Dr. Lad talk about the basics of Ayurveda. These basics deeply resonated with some unknown part of myself. The hair stood up on my arms as a wave of chills swept over me, and I realized that there was a system of medicine that intertwined nutrition, herbal healing, and lifestyle choices to enable us to live harmonious, healthy lives. At that moment, I had no idea exactly what I would do with Ayurveda, but was certain I wanted to learn more.

While I have always found the practical side of Ayurveda its most understandable and, perhaps, useful aspect, I have come to acknowledge the importance of its underlying philosophy. Examining the principles behind the system is essential to understanding its depth, reasoning, and wisdom. After years of tutoring hundreds of students in Ayurveda in a distance-learning program, I find myself continually saying to them, "Just hang on! The philosophical background and all the technical information will become clearer as time progresses and you move forward in your understanding." With that being said, here are the basics to wet your feet.

Ayurveda: The Basic Principles

Ayurveda is a comprehensive natural healing system that covers all aspects of our being: mental, physical, emotional, and spiritual. The term *Ayurveda* combines two Sanskrit words, *ayur* meaning life and longevity, and *veda* meaning wisdom, science, and knowledge. So *Ayurveda* can mean "the science/knowledge of life/longevity."

Ayurveda is the traditional medicine of India; its roots go back over five thousand years. Often referred to as the "mother of all healing," Ayurveda may be the oldest healthcare system in the world. It is not only a medical system, but also a framework for living a healthy life with a peaceful mind.

Thousands of years ago, *rishis*, or "seers," immersed in their meditations, received information and instructions about truth. From these insights they compiled the Vedas, or ancient scriptural texts from India. There are four Vedas today; two of them, the Rig Veda and Atharva Veda, give detailed information about healing, longevity, and surgery. Ayurveda is rooted in these scriptures. The Sankhya philosophy of creation also arose from these ancient scriptural roots. This philosophy is based on two fundamental principles: spirit, or purusha, and matter, or prakruti. It is the union of spirit and matter that produces all things, including the five elements. Both Ayurveda and yoga are based on this Sankhya philosophy.

The Physical Body: Elements and Doshas

The concept of the five elements is at the heart of Ayurveda, and provides a foundation for understanding yourself and the world around you. Energy manifests into five basic principles or elements: ether (space), air, fire, water, and earth. These elements are the building blocks from which the universe manifests and functions.

Earth is the solid state of matter, representing structure and stability.

Water is the liquid state of matter, representing cohesion and flux.

Fire is the transformative state, representing the transition from solid to liquid to gas.

Air is the gaseous state of matter, representing movement.

Ether (or space) is the field of expression from which all is manifested and into which all returns.

Water is an ideal example for understanding all the elements in one substance. Ice is the solid form of water, representing the earth element. Heat or fire causes ice to melt, creating water. Heat also creates steam, which represents the air element. When the steam disappears, it goes into space or ether. This example embodies the interconnectedness within the web of life, all substances visible and invisible in the universe. The five elements are present in matter and arise from energy, demonstrating that energy and matter are interchangeable.

In our body, the five elements produce *dhatus* (structural tissues), *malas* (waste products), and *doshas*. The doshas govern all biological, physiological, and psychological functions of our organism. The word *dosha* means fault, defect, or imperfection, because the doshas are what go out of balance.

The three doshas are *Vata, Pitta,* and *Kapha.* Each dosha is comprised of two elements.

Vata, or "wind," is manifested from air and ether (space).

Pitta, or "bile," is manifested from fire and water.

Kapha, or "phlegm," is manifested from water and earth.

The three doshas can be recognized by their qualities:

- Vata is dry, light, cold, rough, subtle, mobile, clear, and dispersing.
- Pitta is oily, sharp (as in penetrating), hot, light (as in bright), mobile (as in spreading), liquid, and malodorous.
- Kapha is heavy, slow, cold, oily (as in wet or unctuous), slimy (as in gelatinous), dense, soft, static (as in stable), cloudy, hard, and gross (as in the opposite of subtle).

VATA

Vata is the principle of activity governing all movements in the body via the nervous system: breathing, thinking, muscle movement, swallowing, bowel movements, urination, menstruation, and childbirth. Vata is the life force itself, and therefore very powerful. It is the most difficult dosha to keep in balance. Vata is present throughout the body but is predominant in several areas: the bones, colon, brain, lower pelvic abdominal girdle, thighs, ears, hair, and skin. Its primary site is the colon.

Vata types (people in whom Vata is the strongest dosha) usually have a thin body-frame and dry skin, hair, and nails. Their body temperature tends to run cool, creating cold hands and feet. As Vata's energy is often erratic in nature, Vata types will have bursts of energy followed by fatigue. Their digestion tends to be very sensitive, and they tend to be light sleepers.

On the positive side, Vata types are often enthusiastic, creative, flexible, perceptive, and entertaining. They are often great artists, writers, and researchers. When unbalanced, they tend to experience conditions such as constipation, insomnia, weight loss, and arthritis, and become anxious, restless, and indecisive.

Vata is balanced by the following basic lifestyle habits:

- keeping a regular routine for eating, sleeping, working, and leisure time
- staying warm and calm
- receiving plenty of rest and going to bed early
- favoring soothing music
- choosing warm colors for your clothing and environment, such as earth colors, pastels, browns, and warm yellows

Vata is also balanced by the following dietary guidelines:

- eating ample amounts of warm and moist foods, such as porridges and stews
- using mild spices such as cardamom, ginger, cinnamon, basil, and oregano
- generously eating healthy fats and oils such as ghee, sesame oil, and avocado
- avoiding cold, frozen, and raw foods

PITTA

Pitta governs digestion and transformation of all physical and mental processes, from hunger and thirst to body temperature and comprehension. It rules the radiance of the skin and regulates enzymatic and hormonal activity. In the physical body, Pitta resides in the small intestine, stomach, liver, gall bladder, spleen, sweat, blood, sebaceous glands, gray matter of the brain, eyes, skin, and subcutaneous fat. Its main site is in the small intestine.

Pitta types tend to have a fiery nature, are usually medium size and weight, have a warm body temperature, and tend to have strong digestion and can eat almost anything. Pitta types often sleep soundly for short periods of time, and have a strong sex drive. When in balance, they tend to have abundant energy, a beautiful complexion, and strong appetites. When out of balance they often suffer from acid indigestion, inflammation, and skin rashes.

Pitta types are intelligent, organized, precise, and incredibly focused. They are often great teachers, leaders, and decision-makers. However, they have a tendency to become critical, short-tempered, overly competitive, and angry.

Pitta is balanced by the following basic lifestyle habits:

- practicing moderation in all endeavors
- trying not to create unnecessary pressures and stress
- avoiding exposure to excessive heat, such as in saunas or being outside in the heat of the day
- practicing soothing yoga and meditation and exercise during the cooler times of day
- choosing cool colors for your clothing and environment, such as white, green, blue, and silver

Pitta is also balanced by the following dietary guidelines:

- eating cool, soothing foods, such as cucumber, coconut, and melons
- favoring cooling spices such as cilantro, fennel, coriander, and mint
- using olive, coconut, and sunflower oils
- avoiding hot, spicy, salty, oily, and sour foods

KAPHA

Kapha is responsible for stability and structure in the body and mind. The earth and water elements lay a solid foundation for all other things to develop. It is the principle that holds the cells together and forms the muscles, fat, bone, and organs.

Kapha provides moisture to the skin, lubricates joints, and heals wounds. It dwells in the stomach, lungs, throat, sinus, nose, tongue and mouth, white matter and meninges of the brain, pancreas, lymph nodes, plasma, and mastic tissue. Its main site is in the stomach.

A large body-frame with a strong build and excellent stamina are key characteristics of Kapha types. They tend to have thick hair, large eyes, and smooth, radiant skin. They are often sound sleepers and will oversleep if left without an alarm clock. When Kapha is in excess, everything becomes heavy and filled with water, fat, and other bodily fluids. Kapha types may become overweight, lethargic, depressed, and diabetic.

Kapha types tend to be calm, loving, consistent, patient, and compassionate. They like the relaxed life and are good at it! They are often great counselors and nurses, and can handle stressful work situations that involve caring for others. However, they can become stubborn, slow, lazy, and resistant to change.

Kapha is balanced by the following basic lifestyle habits:

- focusing on stimulation and invigoration
- varying your routine
- keeping active and getting plenty of exercise
- staying warm and avoiding dampness
- favoring warm and bright colors for your clothing and environment, such as yellow, orange, and red

Kapha is also balanced by the following dietary guidelines:

- generously using spices, such as ginger, pepper, and mustard
- using small amounts of extra-virgin olive oil and sunflower oil
- minimizing intake of dairy and wheat, and heavy, oily, and fatty foods; using small amounts of low-fat, non-fat, or goat dairy products
- drinking hot ginger tea with meals to stimulate digestion

Complete lists of foods to favor and avoid for each dosha can be found in appendix 2, "Food Guidelines."

Your Unique Constitution: Prakruti and Vikruti

An essential element of Ayurveda is determining your body type or individual constitution—your prakruti. This is the genetic predisposition that, throughout life, governs your inherent strengths, weaknesses, characteristics, and tendencies. It is determined at the moment of conception from your parents' combination of the three doshas. Two children with the same parents can have very different constitutions based on ratios of the three doshas present in their parents at the time of conception. Your prakruti is fixed and remains constant throughout the course of your life, just as the frame of your body won't change.

Your prakruti is seen as a unique combination of the three doshas. There are seven basic constitutional types:

1. Vata
2. Pitta
3. Kapha
4. Vata Pitta or Pitta Vata
5. Vata Kapha or Kapha Vata
6. Pitta Kapha or Kapha Pitta
7. Vata-Pitta-Kapha

In some people one dosha is solidly predominant; the dosha is so strong that it completely overtakes the other two. Dual types exist when one dosha dominates, but another significantly influences a person's life as well; for example, Vata Pitta or Vata Kapha. Dual types are more common than single or tridoshic types. Tridoshic types are either incredibly well balanced, so one dosha doesn't dominate, or all the doshas are imbalanced, which makes treating tridoshic types all the more difficult.

I was fascinated the first time I did an Ayurvedic self-assessment. I thought I understood myself before, but afterward I could see the intelligence of this system shine through. I realized aspects of myself that are part of how I came into this world and affect elements of who I am, like my temperament and appetite. This gave me insight into how I could make small choices every day to feel healthier and happier. Later down the road, I had a professional consultation that affirmed what I had discovered about myself, but also helped me to fine-tune my diet and lifestyle to create a deeper sense of wellness.

After understanding your prakruti, it is essential to look at your current changeable state of health, your vikruti. It is how you have been feeling recently and is often different than your prakruti. Knowing your current vikruti shows you where to focus in order to bring yourself back into balance.

Dosha Self-Assessment

For this exercise, go through the dosha chart two times. The first time, circle your choices based on what has been most consistent for the majority of your life (your prakruti). Then go back with a different-colored pen and circle choices that reflect how you feel right now (your vikruti). If more than one quality is applicable, circle all that apply. It helps to be as honest as possible or have someone close to you fill out the chart for you.

Remember that your goal is to recognize how the characteristics of each dosha express themselves in you. Identifying your body type allows you to choose an appropriate diet and lifestyle to nurture your unique nature, ward off future imbalance, and prevent disease. When you finish, add up the numbers of circles from each column and write the totals in the spaces indicated.

Dosha Chart

	VATA	PITTA	KAPHA
HAIR	dry, thin, dark, frizzy	straight, fine, reddish, oily	oily, wavy, thick, blond, black or dark brown
EYES	small, dry, brown, gray, black, nervous	almond shaped, hazel, penetrating, green, light brown, sensitive to light	big, thick eyelashes, blue, black, dark brown, calm
NAILS	dry, ridged, break easily	clear, well formed, pink, lustrous	square, white, even, thick
LIPS	black/brown color, dry, cracked	red, yellowish, inflamed	oily, smooth, pale, whitish
BODY-FRAME	thin, very tall or very short, irregular	medium, proportionate	broad, heavy, evenly proportioned
SKIN	dry, rough, tans easily, cool, dark	warm, light, reddish, oily, sunburns easily	cool, oily, tans easily, pale, white

Dosha Chart, continued

	VATA	PITTA	KAPHA
JOINTS	cracking, cold	medium or moderately sized, inflamed	lubricated, large
TEETH	big, thin gums, stick out	tender gums, medium size, soft	strong gums, healthy, white
WEIGHT GAIN	hard to gain, easy to lose	easy to gain, easy to lose	easy to gain, hard to lose
APPETITE	variable, scanty	good, intense	consistent
THIRST	variable	excessive	scanty
ELIMINATION	dry, hard, constipated	soft, oily, loose	thick, heavy, slow
STAMINA	poor, exertive	moderate, driven	excellent but lethargic
SWEAT	scanty	profuse	moderate
SLEEP	interrupted, variable	moderate, light	deep, long
TEMPERAMENT	perceptive, indecisive, nervous, unpredictable,	intelligent, successful, irritable, aggressive, jealous	stable, calm, attached, stubborn, greedy
MEMORY	learns quickly, forgets quickly	learns quickly, forgets slowly	learns slowly, forgets slowly
SPEECH	talkative, fast, erratic	decisive, articulate	slow, cautious
DREAMS	flying, jumping, running	fiery, intense, violent	watery, swimming, romantic
SEXUALITY	cold, variable	hot, intense	warm, enduring
FINANCIAL	poor, spends on trifles	spends money on luxuries	rich, saves money well

LIFELONG (PRAKRUTI)	Vata	Pitta	Kapha
CURRENT (VIKRUTI)	Vata	Pitta	Kapha

The dosha self-assessment can help you understand the ratios of doshas in your prakruti and vikruti. If your prakruti and vikruti are about the same, then you would follow a program (diet, lifestyle, etc.) for your strongest dosha. For example, if your vikruti shows Vata higher than in your prakruti, then you would follow a Vata-reducing program, which would include following a diet and lifestyle to balance Vata dosha.

- Which dosha is the highest number in your prakruti?
- Which dosha is the highest number in your vikruti?
- Which diet and lifestyle (Vata, Pitta, or Kapha) are best for you? ◗

The Subtle Body: Prana, Tejas, and Ojas

The three doshas also have subtle, energetic counterparts, referred to as "three vital essences," called *prana*, *tejas*, and *ojas*. Prana, or the life force, is the pure essence of Vata dosha and the ether element. It is a chief force guiding the intelligence behind all mental and physical processes. Tejas (pronounced tey-jas), or "inner radiance," is the pure essence of Pitta dosha and the fire element. This is the subtle energy through which we digest and transform everything we take in: food, liquids, impressions, thoughts, and actions. Ojas (pronounced oh-jas), or "primal vigor," is the pure essence of Kapha dosha and the water element. Ojas governs immunity and vitality, and helps to maintain natural resistance.

The most important of these vital essences to develop, especially when pregnant, is ojas, because it is the essential vitality that gives endurance and strength, and creates a buffer when harsh winds blow. It is said that abundant ojas in the mother creates love and compassion that she passes on to her baby. Increasing ojas is not just about building it up, but also about not losing or wasting it. Ojas is lost by:

- stress
- lack of sleep
- poor digestion
- overwork
- excessive anger, grief, and worrying
- too much sex

Ojas can be strengthened and replenished by:

- following a diet and lifestyle appropriate to your constitution;
- eating nourishing foods, which include almonds, walnuts, honey, saffron, ghee, whole grains, certain legumes (like mung beans), root vegetables, and dairy products (particularly warm, spiced milk—see chapter 7, page 89);
- spending time in nature;
- sleeping soundly;

- taking a break from electronics and media stimulation;
- practicing meditation, chanting, and certain breathing exercises (pranayama);
- taking rejuvenating herbs such as amalaki (*Emblica officinalis*), the primary ingredient in the Ayurvedic herbal jelly called *chyavanprash*, which can be helpful for all body types; shatavari; and ashwagandha (during pregnancy, use only under the guidance of an Ayurvedic practitioner or herbalist).

Taking a relaxing vacation does wonders for ojas. Spending time away from computers, telephones, televisions, and your daily demands allows your nervous system to relax deeply and rejuvenate. Have you ever noticed a lustrous glow on people when they return from a restful holiday in nature? That is ojas.

EXERCISE

Assessing Your Ojas

Look at the ojas assessment chart and see if you have characteristics of an optimal state of ojas or signs and symptoms of a suboptimal state. Circle what is correct for you.

Ojas Assessment

	OJAS
CHARACTERISTICS OF OPTIMAL STATE	strong immunity
	happy and cheerful disposition
	loving and compassionate
	excellent strength and endurance
	good retention of knowledge
	glowing skin
	lustrous eyes
	shiny hair
	good sexual endurance
	calm and content

Ojas Assessment, continued

	OJAS
SIGNS AND SYMPTOMS OF SUBOPTIMAL STATE	extreme fatigue
	lack of zest for life
	lack of confidence
	chronic Vata disorders
	thin, emaciated body
	poor mental ability
	lack of clarity
	dehydration, lack of luster
	susceptibility to infections
	hyperactive mind
	muscle wasting

When you are finished, ask yourself:

- Is my ojas in an optimal or suboptimal state?
- What is one thing I can do to build up my ojas? 🌢

The Mental Body: Sattva, Rajas, and Tamas

The nature and qualities of the mind are referred to as the mental constitution, or *manas prakruti*. Ayurveda examines the psychological traits and propensities innate to each of us. They are part of our genetics and are formed at the time of fertilization. Just as the physical body is viewed in terms of the doshas, the mind is viewed in terms of three *gunas*, called *sattva*, *rajas*, and *tamas*. Each of these comprises a set of qualities.

Sattva is seen in the qualities of clarity, alertness, compassion, balance, love, and awareness.

Rajas is seen in the qualities of movement, agitation, self-centeredness, willfulness, and ego.

Tamas is seen in the qualities of inertia, darkness, heaviness, dullness, and sadness.

Almost everyone has each quality or guna present, but in different proportions. The beautiful aspect about your mental constitution is that it is not permanent and can change with awareness, action, and association. You may enter life with more rajasic or tamasic tendencies, or have some psychological problems, yet you may also have the ability to deal with them. However, you can evolve and change from rajas or tamas into sattva through meditation, prayer, and serving others, for example. This awareness can help with spiritual growth and peace of mind. One of the primary goals of yoga and Ayurveda is to cultivate more sattva.

A few years ago I revisited my guna chart to prepare for a class I was teaching, and discovered something about myself. In the section on forgiveness I reread the categories: sattva, forgives freely; rajas, forgives with effort; and tamas, holds a grudge. It brought to light a situation where I was holding a grudge against someone who had been a close friend and did something hurtful to me. After reading these words in black and white, I realized that: (1) she did not purposely harm me, but was acting from a place of discontentment; (2) I wanted to be able to forgive freely; and (3) I did not want to be tamasic! This new awareness helped me to let go of the grudge, and subsequently I felt much happier inside.

Ayurveda always emphasizes sattva as the highest state—clear, pure, and divine. Sattva allows perception to occur, brings about the inward movement of consciousness, and unifies the mind and heart. Sattva is also seen as a balance of the positive expressions of all three gunas.

A very highly sattvic nature is rare and often indicates a saint or sage. When I think of someone purely sattvic, I envision a yogi living in a cave up in the mountains, wearing all white, meditating all day, and surviving on fruits and roots. While this is a beautiful image, it is not reality for most of us living in the world. Here in the West, a sattvic person might be someone who is considered of high moral character. Generally, the qualities of sattva are sorely lacking in our busy and often frantic modern society.

EXERCISE

Understanding Your Mind

When you examine how the gunas are present in your mind and in your life, you can see your mental and spiritual state and inclinations. The mental constitution (guna) chart will help you grasp your mental makeup.

Circle the traits that best represent you, and then have someone you know well answer for you. Do not judge yourself! The majority of your answers will probably fall in the middle category or rajasic area, as this is the main spiritual state in our culture today. Again, the purpose of this exercise is to elucidate where you are and to point you toward where you might like to be.

Mental Constitution (Guna) Chart

	SATTVA	RAJAS	TAMAS
TRUTHFULNESS	always	most of the time	rarely
PEACE OF MIND	always	mostly	rarely
SPIRITUAL STUDY	daily	occasionally	never
MEDITATION	daily	occasionally	never
PRAYER	daily	occasionally	never
SELFLESS SERVICE	often	occasionally	rarely
CREATIVITY	high	moderate	low
WILLPOWER	strong	variable	weak
MEMORY	good	moderate	poor
CONCENTRATION	very clear	hyperactive	cloudy
FORGIVENESS	forgives easily	with effort	holds grudges
PRIDE	modest	some ego	vain
LOVE	unconditional universal	personal	lacking in love
RELATIONSHIPS	harmonious	passionate	disturbed
SPEECH	peaceful and calm	agitated	dull
HYGIENE	high	moderate	low
WORK	noble, selfless	for personal goals	lazy, sluggish
DIET	vegetarian	some meat	heavy meat diet
DRUGS/ALCOHOL/STIMULANTS	never	occasionally	frequently
CONTROL OF SENSES	good	moderate	weak
ADDICTIVE BEHAVIOR	never	occasionally	frequently
ANGER	hardly ever	sometimes	frequently
FEAR	hardly ever	sometimes	frequently
DEPRESSION	hardly ever	sometimes	frequently
TOTAL			

- Were you surprised by what you learned about yourself from this exercise?
- What areas were sensitive spots for you, and why?
- How can you take steps to move toward more sattva in your life? ◊

This chapter has given you a context for understanding the larger picture of Ayurveda, which can help you to see yourself (and the world) in a new light. Hopefully, you now know a little more about yourself.

Promoting positive health and preventing disease are foundational aspects of Ayurveda. By understanding your unique makeup, you can choose elemental pieces of your puzzle to promote the healthiest version of yourself: balanced, energized, happy (with increased vitality). These qualities are invaluable in everyday life, and especially in pregnancy. It is best to begin making small changes that can then build into larger ones, as a complete overhaul can be difficult to sustain and can potentially backfire. Check out the resources section at the back of the book for recommended readings if you are curious to learn more about the philosophical foundations of Ayurveda. Or simply proceed with the rest of the book and extract what is helpful for you.

2

The Complete Practice of Yoga

*In the practice of Yoga one can emphasize the body, the mind or the self
and hence the effort can never be fruitless.*
KRISHNAMACHARYA

Fundamental Principles of Prenatal Yoga

Whether you are a seasoned practitioner or have never practiced a posture in your life, yoga can impart a deep sense of tranquility and comfort through the ebbs and flows of your pregnancy. Yoga strengthens, refines, and stabilizes your body, breath, and mind. Moreover, prenatal yoga can help you soften and yield to the monumental process that is happening within. This acquiescence can cultivate an overarching feeling that your pregnancy is evolving the way Mother Nature intends.

Each trimester brings different gifts and challenges to each woman. One of the blessings of yoga is learning how to tune in and bring awareness to the changing states of your body, breath, and mind. By creating time and space to reflect on where you are and where you would like to be, you can set intentions for bringing yourself back into balance.

My personal yoga practices shifted throughout the course of my pregnancies. When I was pregnant with my son, the first trimester nausea prevented me from practicing almost any asanas (yoga postures). I focused solely on pranayama (breathing practices) and meditation to balance my emotions and get through that uncomfortable time. As the nausea subsided in the second trimester, yoga helped strengthen my back, and pranayama helped me settle down at night so I could relax deeply and sleep soundly. My third trimester practices were invigorating so I could keep my energy strong and create a sense of lightness in my expanding body. I used this time to refine pranayama, which allowed me to go deeper in meditation and feel more prepared and peaceful approaching birth.

The primary purpose of prenatal yoga is to support a pregnant woman's whole being. Many often think of yoga as an attempt to get into complex postures. Moving beyond this limited idea of yoga can help you see that the function of postures and practices—how they affect your body, breath, and mind—is more important than their appearance. A complete practice of yoga includes:

- movement
- breathing exercises
- meditation
- possibly chanting or sound exercises
- adopting universal ideas for a harmonious life based on the underlying philosophy of yoga

According to T. K. V. Desikachar, true mastery of yoga is really measured by "how it influences our day-to-day living, how it enhances our relationships, how it promotes clarity and peace of mind."

Your attitude or intention as a *yogini* (a woman who practices yoga) is vital and sets the tone for what you receive from yoga. If you have been practicing yoga for some time and are newly pregnant, you will see how aspects of yoga are tailored for pregnancy. By practicing yoga appropriately for your stage of pregnancy, both you and your growing baby will benefit.

Each woman has her own unique experience of how yoga affects her. Frequently, women find that doing yoga postures increases circulation, flexibility, stamina, and balance; strengthens back muscles; increases mental alertness and concentration; improves digestion, uplifts energy, and reduces fatigue and stress. Many feel more relaxed and peaceful after practicing. Research suggests that prenatal yoga can also improve sleep;

relieve lower back pain; reduce nausea, headaches, and shortness of breath; and lower the risk of preterm labor and pregnancy-induced hypertension.

Many pregnant women find that yoga is a way to connect with their baby and is an opportunity to do something special to honor their pregnancy. Prenatal yoga helps a woman to prepare for a peaceful and natural birth, to develop self-confidence and trust, and to feel comfortable with a changing body, wavering emotions, and other common challenges.

If you choose to work with a yoga teacher privately, she can develop a personalized yoga practice specifically designed for you and your stage of pregnancy, taking into account your uniqueness (body, breath, and mind) while also considering your work, daily activities, and responsibilities.

Different practices for the morning and evening can help address specific concerns. Morning yoga practices can increase energy, dispel morning sickness, enhance alertness, and help prepare for a busy day. An evening yoga practice can help release stress from the day, improve circulation, and promote relaxation. See the resources section for a directory of yoga teachers trained in adapting yoga to individual situations.

Group prenatal yoga classes are a more affordable option for many and are also a wonderful way to connect with other like-minded pregnant women. The camaraderie, support, and fun that develop out of these classes can uplift and enrich your experience of being pregnant. Find a teacher whose style resonates with you, and who is also adequately trained in prenatal yoga. If you continue to attend regular yoga classes (not specifically prenatal), it is wise to let your teacher know that you are pregnant.

Practicing yoga does not need to be a lengthy, time-consuming activity if your life does not allow for it. Short practices done regularly can be highly effective. Taking a break from your computer for five to ten minutes to stretch and breathe, or spending ten to twenty minutes before bed in relaxing, restorative poses can be very helpful. In a workshop I attended years ago, a master yoga teacher commented that a very busy person who practices for five minutes a day can get just as much benefit as a person who is less busy and practices many hours a day.

When both of my children were babies, I sat in meditation right after they fell asleep for their naps. I propped myself up on a pillow to help straighten my spine, watched my breath, and silently recited a mantra for five minutes. This small span of time felt huge in my busy, hectic day, and served me a thousandfold. I tried to carve out larger blocks of time a few days a week for longer yoga practices, but I always knew that I had these short, daily meditations to sustain me.

Body: Prenatal Yoga Postures (Asanas)

Most prenatal yoga asanas are modified according to a woman's growing belly, which affects her center of gravity, spine, and other body parts and systems (circulatory system, digestive system, joints, and ligaments). Generally, pregnant women should practice all poses with the legs hip-width or wider. For example, many classical poses begin with the feet close together, but in pregnancy, when the hips naturally widen, it is more comfortable to begin with the feet hip-width apart or even a little wider. The wider stance will help women feel a solid base of support and stability, which is of the utmost importance. It is also important to emphasize bending the knees in various postures.

Jumping, deep forward bends, deep back arches, deep twists, and all poses that put pressure on the baby are *contraindicated* during pregnancy. Practicing asanas that involve contracting the abdomen is also to be avoided. It is important *not* to lie flat on the back after the fourth month because the vena cava and femoral arteries can become compressed, which interferes with blood flow to the fetus.

Create a space for yourself in your home that is clean, uncluttered, and quiet. It is best to avoid eating anything heavy within two hours of practice. Loose, comfortable clothes are easiest for movement. You can do yoga on a clean blanket or towel, or you may wish to purchase a yoga mat and other props. Props such as blankets, chairs, and bolsters may be helpful in achieving proper positioning and greater comfort within an asana. Some women prefer not to use props and naturally work with their changing bodies. Choose what works for you, as both approaches are completely fine. (The resources section includes recommended websites for ordering yoga mats and props.)

Breath: Breathing Practices (Pranayama)

Our body, breath, and mind are interdependent, and prana, our life force and breath, is the energy of movement between them. When prana flows smoothly, all our bodily systems function more efficiently. When it is disturbed or impeded, imbalances arise. Working with our breath brings new awareness, as our state of mind is intimately linked with the quality of prana within our body. This awareness allows us to choose and control our actions and to lessen our reactions.

One of my great yoga teachers always said, "Be kind to your breath and treat it like a friend." I think this is sound advice, as it is especially important to start working with your breath in pregnancy, since it will be your greatest tool in labor. Your breath will help you through contractions by allowing you to deeply let go and relax between each contraction. As you move from pregnancy into motherhood, pranayama can help you cope with stressful situations, increase your energy, access your intuition, relax, and become more peaceful.

Pranayama practices are best begun slowly and gradually, to allow for a full integration. This helps the mind make the transition from one state to another. In pregnancy, it is especially important *not* to do any forceful breathing or retentions of breath. The breathing practices most appropriate are *ujjayi, shitali,* and *nadi shodhana.* All three are explained in detail throughout the book, and can be used freely throughout pregnancy. If you are already accustomed to these practices, there is always room for refinement and building on what you know. Always stop if you feel dizzy, light-headed, or out of breath, and allow a few minutes for the breath to normalize upon completion.

For all of the breathing exercises, take time to find a comfortable sitting position, so you can stay seated for a period of time without becoming stiff or sore. Let the breath lengthen the spine rather than the other way around. Eventually, the breathing techniques will be a seamless entrance into a deeper relationship with your breath.

EXERCISE

Observing the Qualities of Your Breath

The breath is an excellent indicator of your current physical and emotional state of health. By observing your breath, you're taking steps to tune into yourself. New awareness always brings more opportunities for understanding, change, and growth.

For this exercise, just observe your breath. There is no right or wrong way to breathe. Close your eyes and focus on your breathing to tune out any external stimuli. Take four to five breaths. What do you notice? Is your breath:

- flowing smoothly, or shaky with impediments?
- short (under two seconds), or long (over four seconds)?
- slow and deep, or fast paced and superficial?

Take a few more breaths. Notice if:

- your breath is mostly in the chest, down in the belly, or both;
- if your inhalation is longer or shorter than your exhalation. 💧

Mind: Meditation

Many women naturally turn inward during pregnancy and find themselves drawn to quiet and contemplative activities. This is an opportune time to explore the inner limbs (or deeper practices) of yoga, such as meditation. You may find yourself craving stillness and deep relaxation, or maybe you just have awareness that meditation is a healthy endeavor in which to engage your mind.

Meditation is a general term for contemplating or reflecting upon something with a quiet mind. According to the Yoga Sutras (a classical text on the philosophy of yoga), there are three stages of meditation: *dharana*, *dhyana*, and *samadhi*. Each involves a process of focusing and stilling the mind to a new state of awareness.

Many styles of meditation exist, and most begin with choosing a focus or linking to something that is positive and healing. The Sanskrit word *bhavana* means intention, attitude, or focus. Bhavana is used as a tool for meditation as it is immensely powerful and helpful to meditate with an intention. Bhavana also includes visualizations. Selecting a focus for your meditation is an intimate choice. Many people choose to simply focus on their breath. Here are some specific bhavanas, or points of focus, for meditation in pregnancy:

- A feeling of protection or trust in the divine forces in the world.
- The image of a healthy baby growing inside, or a smooth and gentle birth.
- An object from nature, such as the sun at dawn or a bright blooming flower. Or taking it further, you could choose to see a calm mountain lake as representing calm and peacefulness inside yourself.
- An idea such as compassion or kindness, for yourself or another.
- A higher force, a feeling of the Divine or God, or a symbol that represents it, such as Buddha, Ganesha, or Mary.
- The sounds *so hum* or other mantras.

Exercise

Exploring Intentions for Your Meditations

There are ten guided meditations in this book, but there may be times when you want one with a more personal focus. An intention for meditation can be just as unique as you are, especially in your pregnancy. Take a few minutes and explore some ideas for meditations.

- Is there something healing and inspiring you would like to link to—perhaps something from the natural world or a positive quality?
- Are there sounds that resonate with you or that a teacher has taught you?
- What is supportive that you would like to visualize for yourself and/or your family?

Make your own list of bhavanas for meditation. Keep the list near where you practice yoga. Make a commitment to meditate with a bhavana for the next week and observe how you feel afterward. ◊

Personally, I found visualizations and mantra meditation helpful in my pregnancies. Visualizations helped to create pictures of what I envisioned for my babies and myself. I also chose sacred sounds that represented qualities I wanted to draw toward me. When I teach prenatal yoga, I always include a bhavana for meditation at the end of class. Women are free to focus on the idea or not, but at least they have guidance on how to go deeper into their meditation practice.

Meditation in pregnancy can help reduce stress and alleviate many physiological symptoms, such as morning sickness and high blood pressure. Pregnancy meditations especially help to increase your connection with your baby and to feel more empowered. When you feel peaceful and relaxed, you can communicate these feelings to your baby. A regular meditation practice can help prepare for birth as you learn to consciously relax, focus, work with the breath, and find your strength within.

Meditation comes easiest after movement (asana) and breathing (pranayama). Asana opens, stretches, and prepares the body to sit at ease, while pranayama helps to stabilize the breath. These practices support and enhance each other.

Once you are prepared and ready to meditate, the mind consciously and continuously focuses on the chosen idea, intention, or your breath, and other distracting thoughts naturally dissipate as you seamlessly fall into an expanded state of awareness. This stage is called dhyana. It may be more difficult to enter this state than it seems. Don't get discouraged! Everyone's mind naturally wanders. Just keep bringing your awareness back to your breath or chosen point of focus. Even meditating for one minute is beneficial.

Focal Points for Practice by Trimester

In part 2 of this book, movement, breathing, sound, and meditation practices are mapped out for the course of your entire pregnancy. The following, however, is a brief summary of what to expect.

FIRST TRIMESTER

The first trimester is a very delicate phase and does not lend itself to following an asana practice guided by a book. So the first trimester practices outlined in part 2 include breathing, sound, and meditation, but no asana practices.

If you have never practiced yoga before, it is best to wait until after the first trimester to begin practicing asanas. The fetus needs good implantation, which occurs during this time. Any new movements or exercise programs, including yoga, should wait until after the pregnancy is established.

If you were practicing yoga before becoming pregnant, now is the time to modify your practice and tone it down, like switching from running to fast walking. You want to work gently on strengthening your back, and begin to modify all asanas by taking your feet hip width apart or wider. If you practiced inversions regularly before, such as a headstand, you can continue if it feels right and as long as you are not contracting the abdomen getting into or out of the pose. If you notice any spotting or cramping or feel fatigued after practicing yoga, simply stop and rest. If you are working privately with a teacher, she or he can guide you in a very gentle, safe, first trimester practice.

Any woman with a challenging obstetrical history, such as previous miscarriage(s), abortion(s), difficulty conceiving, or loss of a child, may feel especially vulnerable during the first trimester. Extra care and caution is natural and warranted. Adopting an attitude or bhavana of "protection" can be helpful in your yoga practice.

During the first trimester, many women experience nausea and vomiting (often referred to as NVP), which can affect a woman's interest in and ability to practice yoga. If this is relevant for you, do very gentle yoga postures that do not involve forward movements, or spend your time in pranayama and meditation, which are especially helpful for NVP.

SECOND TRIMESTER

The beginning of the second trimester, as your energy picks up, is an excellent time to dive into the movement aspect of a yoga practice.

In part 2, the fourth month's practice begins with a prenatal asana sequence that can serve as a base movement practice for your pregnancy. Each subsequent month has a different sequence connected to that month's theme, with some of the basic poses from month four and new poses as well. The second and third trimesters have complete practices of movement, breath, sound, and meditation. They are properly designed with counterposes and the correct order of practice, so they are best followed as is. If you want to spend more time in a particular posture or in meditation, please do. Some of the practices may seem basic to the seasoned yogini, but stay open to their subtleties and gifts.

In general, postures that encourage opening the pelvis are invaluable. They increase mobility in the hip and pelvic joints while strengthening and stretching the pelvic floor and perineal area. Pelvic opening postures practiced regularly can facilitate greater comfort as pregnancy progresses, and possibly an easier childbirth.

Balance poses are excellent for building strength in the legs, increasing circulation, improving coordination, and developing stability. With regular practice, you will feel strength and stability not only in your body but also in your daily life. The postures can help you move with grace and a sense of fluid stability through all activities in your day, and help to avoid accidents and injuries.

Mild chest-opening asanas are wonderful to help compensate for the weight of new breast tissue and strain on the back. Supported restorative poses also feel heavenly, and allow the body to rest deeply, unwind, and release.

If you have regularly practiced inversions, it is best to stop by the end of the fifth month. Adopting an attitude, or bhavana, of "no worry" can be helpful in your yoga practice. You can also visualize whatever you wish for yourself, your growing baby, and evolving family.

THIRD TRIMESTER

Many of the same focal points from the first and second trimesters are carried into the third. The asanas will continue to be modified to an even greater degree, and at this time, the use of props can be very helpful. Protecting the joints, maintaining balance, reestablishing proper alignment of the spine, and increasing circulation are crucial focal points for asana practice. Asana can help you feel more comfortable in your body, while pranayama and chanting can relax the nervous system and help prepare for the challenges of labor.

It's important to try to stay positive so you can enjoy the end of pregnancy and maintain an optimistic attitude for a good birth. It may be helpful to remind yourself "I am strong and confident enough to handle whatever comes my way."

The Three Doshas and Yoga Practice

You can further refine and tailor the practice of yoga by integrating the principles of Ayurveda, mainly the three doshas. In chapter 1, you evaluated yourself in terms of the three doshas. You determined your genetic constitution (prakruti) and your current state (vikruti). Your vikruti will inevitably be colored by your pregnancy. With awareness of which dosha is out of balance, you can follow general guidelines for harmonizing that dosha during your yoga practice.

VATA

Vata types are often attracted to yoga practices that involve quick movement, even though this could aggravate them. Vatas are open to change and enjoy lots of activity. For those with a predominantly Vata constitution or others who are feeling a Vata imbalance due to whatever cause (such as the season, wrong diet, or travel), practice with the following emphasis:

- Let your practice be gentle and soothing.
- Slow down.
- Keep your energy even, firm, and constant.
- Pay extra attention to your breath. Let the breath be deep, calm, and strong.
- Moderate your enthusiasm and try to sustain it.
- Try to stay in the moment.

PITTA

Pitta types are often attracted to very athletic forms of yoga as a means for developing their physique and challenging themselves. They also enjoy meditation and practices that work on the mind. For those with a predominantly Pitta constitution or who are feeling a Pitta imbalance due to whatever cause (such as the season, wrong diet, or pressure at work), practice with the following emphasis:

- Keep your body, breath, and energy cool, receptive, and relaxed.
  Do not overheat.
- Soften.
- Try to be aware and receptive, instead of competitive and critical.
- Relax your jaw and other areas that hold tension in your body.
- Practice asana in a surrendering manner.

KAPHA

Kapha types tend to be drawn to devotional practices such as chanting and prayer. Asana practice can be more difficult because it requires effort. For those with a predominantly Kapha constitution or who are feeling a Kapha imbalance due to whatever cause (such as the season, wrong diet, or feeling lethargic), practice with the following emphasis:

- Warm up properly before practice, and then do asanas at a
  faster pace.
- Challenge yourself by staying in a pose longer or practicing longer
  than usual.
- Pay extra attention to keeping the mind wakeful, enthusiastic,
  and engaged.
- Keep moving and bring a sense of lightness to the body.

An understanding of Ayurvedic principles can change the way you perceive yourself and others. Since I began my studies over fifteen years ago, I am constantly observing the doshas in action, whether I want to or not. I notice other people's constitutions when I'm shopping at the grocery store or picking my children up at school. When I'm teaching yoga, I've found that an Ayurvedic perspective is especially helpful in assisting students to subtly shift some aspect of their practice. I almost always notice a Pitta woman clenching her jaw or comparing her form to others. I will either make a general comment to the whole class based on my observation, or guide her specifically toward balance.

In my own yoga practice, I notice how the time of year influences how the doshas express themselves. For example, in late winter I notice Kapha creeping up on me and I feel slow, heavy, and unfocused. When I catch this happening, I make an extra effort to engage my mind with my breath and to keep my practice active. In the fall, when Vata becomes aggravated naturally, I need to pay more attention to calming the breath and moving slower to keep Vata balanced.

EXERCISE

Observing the Doshas at Play in Your Yoga

The next time you are practicing yoga asanas, either at home or in a class, pay extra attention to the general qualities of the doshas.

- Do you notice characteristics of one dosha dominating you? Which one?
- Try to incorporate the foregoing ideas for balance when you notice something. Then what do you observe?
- Can you take other steps to balance the imbalanced dosha in different areas of your life, such as diet or lifestyle? Does it reflect when you practice yoga again? ◉

Nourishing Diet

The essence of food taken by the mother is divided into three parts—one nourishes her,
the other promotes her breast milk and the third portion nourishes the fetus.
SUSHRUTA SAMHITA

In the early weeks of my first pregnancy, I was eagerly searching for Ayurvedic guidance on what to eat. I thought the five-thousand-year-old system that had brought balance to so many areas of my life and my clients' lives must have some insights to share about diet and pregnancy. When I could not find an authoritative, modern book on Ayurveda and pregnancy, I dove into the classical texts to dig up the knowledge right from its source.

I knew I was not going to find information on how many grams of protein to eat or how much folic acid to consume, but I was fascinated to discover that the texts' ancient guidelines were as applicable to life today as centuries ago. The texts describe what to eat in terms of qualities or attributes of foods. They said the main qualities of foods in pregnancy should be sweet, unctuous, liquid, and "prepared with appetizers."

Sweet refers to one of the six tastes of Ayurveda that is the dominant taste in all forms of nourishment. It is made from the earth and water elements. Sweet is the sweet taste of whole grains, root vegetables, milk, and fresh fruits, not necessarily sugary sweet. The sweet quality of food builds all the bodily tissues and helps to maintain the health of the mother and baby. It gives strength, energy, vitality, and longevity.

Unctuous describes foods of an oily nature, from healthy fats and healthy oils such as avocados, ghee, and extra-virgin olive oil. This quality helps to lubricate the joints, connective tissues, and digestive tract, and promotes strength and protection.

Liquid refers to moist, soupy foods such as porridges and stews, which are generally easy to digest. This ensures you are receiving enough fluids to support the body's expanding blood volume, and helps you to stay hydrated.

Prepared with appetizers alludes to foods prepared with spices and salt to create tasty food that is easy to digest, absorb, and assimilate. It is best if everything a woman experiences during pregnancy is pleasant and delightful, including eating!

Ayurvedic texts also remind us that foods that are hot, spicy, very salty, deep-fried, or that contain large amounts of sugar will not only be difficult to digest, but may upset the baby as well.

Sattvic and Ojas-Building Foods

In pregnancy it is especially important to follow your doctor's or midwife's dietary recommendations, such as guidance about which nutrients to emphasize and how many calories to consume. Many foods that are important from an Ayurvedic and yogic perspective also support and enhance any healthy prenatal diet.

In Ayurveda and yoga, it is important to emphasize foods that are sattvic and ojas building. Ojas governs immunity and vitality and helps to maintain natural resistance. Sattva represents the qualities of balance, higher awareness, clarity, and compassion. Foods of these elements are especially nourishing to an expectant mother and her growing baby. They are pure, wholesome, and incredibly nutritious. They include:

- almonds and walnuts
- dates and figs
- honey (but not raw honey, which should be avoided during pregnancy)

- sesame seeds
- fresh fruits and fresh pressed juices
- saffron and cardamom
- fresh ghee (clarified butter), butter, and milk
- fresh coconut
- split mung beans
- whole grains, like wheat, rice, and quinoa
- root vegetables, like yams, carrots, and beets

I remember that when I accentuated sattvic and ojas-building foods in my diet, I felt more balanced, my tummy was happy, my energy was stable, and I knew that I was deeply nourishing myself and my growing baby. Everything that goes into your mouth does not necessarily need to be one of these foods, but try to incorporate them as much as possible. Since some of these ojas-building foods naturally increase the Kapha dosha, those who are Kapha predominant may not need as much as other types.

When Paulina was sixteen weeks pregnant, she came to see me for guidance on treating constipation and fatigue, among other complaints. One quick look at her diet diary showed that her diet was incredibly lacking in fresh vegetables, fruits, protein, and healthy fats—all crucial components of a balanced prenatal diet. After a simple dietary cleanup, emphasizing ojas-building foods and a few simple lifestyle changes, her energy significantly improved and her constipation disappeared. It's amazing what simple measures can do.

Eating According to Your Body Type

In the first session with each Ayurveda client I see, whether she is pregnant or not, I spend a great deal of time discussing how to eat according to one's body type. Many people mistakenly think that Ayurvedic nutrition is about eating lentils and rice every day. In fact, Ayurvedic nutrition is about understanding yourself: your body, its metabolism, the strength or weakness of your digestive fire, and your tendencies for imbalance. Let these factors, along with the season and what is available locally for you to eat, be the baseline for your diet.

Rejuvenating Ojas Drink

1 handful whole, raw almonds
4 to 5 pitted dates
1 cup water, plus extra for soaking
1 cup milk (whole milk for Vata types, 2% for Pitta types, and skim for Kapha types; almond milk for those who are lactose intolerant)
Pinch of cardamom

Directions

Soak almonds in water overnight. Drain water and peel almonds in the morning. The skins should slide right off.

Place all ingredients in a blender and blend until smooth.

Enjoy. Notice how you feel when you drink it, afterward and even the next day.

Benefits of a Healthy, Well-Balanced Diet

A healthy and well-balanced prenatal diet can prevent:
- anemia
- constipation
- fatigue
- low birth weight
- muscle cramps
- other more serious health problems

Again, in pregnancy it is always important to follow the nutritional recommendations given by your doctor or midwife. You can further enhance your prenatal diet by individualizing it from an Ayurvedic perspective. One of the greatest gifts of Ayurvedic wisdom is direction on how to *eat according to your body type.* Not only will eating this way help you sustain a deep sense of health and stability, but more importantly, it will also help to keep the doshas balanced and prevent all kinds of ailments from developing.

For example, an avocado is an important food for any pregnant woman because it is a good source of heart-healthy unsaturated fat, folate, and fiber, among other nutrients. Since avocados are caloric, heavy, moist, and unctuous, Vata types (who have a hard time gaining weight) could probably eat an entire avocado at a meal, but Pitta types would do best with half, and Kapha types with a quarter. Going one step further, the Vata woman could salt her avocado, the Pitta woman could top it with fresh cilantro, and the Kapha woman could enjoy her portion with lemon and black pepper. This way each type can still receive the benefits and enjoy the yumminess of an avocado in a proportion and with herbs or spices that are appropriate.

If you are unclear about which Ayurvedic diet is best for you, please seek the guidance of a qualified Ayurvedic practitioner. If you are curious to learn more about Ayurvedic cooking and the Ayurvedic view of the nature of foods and their preparations, please read *The Ayurvedic Cookbook* by Amadea Morningstar or *A Life of Balance* by Maya Tiwari. Both books elaborate on these topics and have fantastic recipes. (See the resources section.)

All body types benefit from eating abundant fresh vegetables (especially dark leafy greens and yellow and orange veggies, like carrots and squash, which are naturally high in the vitamins and minerals you need most in pregnancy), fresh fruits, whole grains, ample protein, and healthy, high-quality fats. The food charts in appendix 2, "Food Guidelines," outline details for each body type. Foods closest to their natural state are preferable. Eliminating or minimizing white flours and sugars, artificial sweeteners, low-quality fats, and other "empty" or "junk" foods is also best for moms and babies, regardless of their doshas.

General Dietary Guidelines for Each Dosha

	VATA	PITTA	KAPHA
FAVOR	warm, mildly spiced, moist	cool, non-spicy, sweet	warm, spicy, dry
	sweet, fresh fruits	sweet fruits	astringent fruits such as apples and pomegranates
	cooked veggies	sweet and bitter veggies	bitter and pungent veggies
	grains such as oats, rice, and wheat	grains such as barley, quinoa, and rice	grains such as millet, barley, and buckwheat
	all spices such as cinnamon, ginger, and basil	mild spices such as coriander, mint, and fennel	all spices such as ginger, pepper, and oregano
	small legumes such as split mung and aduki beans	most legumes	most legumes
	most nuts	sunflower and pumpkin seeds	popcorn and chia seeds
	ample amounts of sesame and olive oils, as well as ghee	moderate amounts of sunflower, coconut, and olive oils, as well as ghee	small amounts of corn, sunflower, and olive oils, as well as ghee
AVOID	dry, frozen, cold, astringent	spicy, sour, oily, salty	heavy, fatty, salty, oily
	dried fruits, as well as raw and frozen vegetables	sour fruits and pungent vegetables	sweet or sour fruits, as well as sweet and juicy vegetables
	nightshades such as tomatoes and peppers	fermented foods	most dairy products
	dry, powdered milk	pungent teas	cold foods and drinks

Ayurveda follows the commonsense concept of "like increases like" and "opposites balance each other." For example, if you are feeling especially cold in the winter (Vata quality in Vata season), eating a Popsicle outside in the snow without a jacket will only make you feel colder and aggravated (like increases like). But if you are a Vata type, and you are inside in the winter, bundled up in woolens by the fire, eating warm ginger-squash soup, you will likely feel warm, toasty, and happy (opposites balance).

All the doshas can be examined by their qualities, such as cold/hot, dry/moist, as you saw in chapter 1. Consuming foods with the same qualities as a dosha will increase it, while consuming foods of the opposite qualities will balance it.

Current research is confirming that nourishing a fetus involves more than just what a woman eats in pregnancy: that is, a woman's body composition can affect how well her placenta transfers nutrients to the fetus. This aligns with the Ayurvedic theory of the three doshas. For example, thin women with low amounts of muscle (Vata types) are less able to handle protein than more muscular women. So Vata types do better eating frequent little meals with small amounts of protein in each one. Women who carry large amounts of fat (Kapha types) are often in a constant state of inflammation, which can affect the formation and function of the placenta. It would behoove a Kapha woman to try to eat less fat before pregnancy, decreasing her risk of hypertension or diabetes in pregnancy. When the doshas are in a state of equilibrium, all our health is in a more balanced state. Our diet and lifestyle are shaping the next generation, so the stronger our health is before *and* during pregnancy, the same may be bestowed upon our children.

EXERCISE

What Do the Dosha Guidelines Mean for You?

These general principles are here to get you started. Please refer to the food list in appendix 2 for a complete look at all the foods to favor and to avoid for each constitution. You can also check out the Recommended Reading list for additional books that elaborate on these ideas. After completing the dosha self-assessment in chapter 1, think about your constitution and which diet would be best for you. It is easiest to target one dosha at a time—whichever is most predominant.

- What foods and types of foods are best for you? Which are not so good?
- How does this compare to what you typically eat?
- What would be an ideal meal for your constitution? What would be the worst?

Keep in mind that certain qualities can vary widely depending on the food. For example, both corn and cayenne pepper are considered warming and Pitta aggravating. Yet corn is only slightly warming, while cayenne pepper is extremely hot. Therefore a Pitta-reducing diet should completely avoid something like cayenne pepper, but corn is okay in moderation.

Digestion

Awareness of how you are digesting food is critical in Ayurveda, since many imbalances arise from poor digestion. *Agni*, the digestive fire, is the force within the body that transforms food into energy through its role in digestion, absorption, and assimilation of food. The digestive agni can be viewed as a small fire burning inside the body. You need to tend the fire, feed it appropriately sized kindling first, then larger wood, and stoke it regularly to maintain the flame. When the fire burns with a healthy flame and glow, food is digested well and at the proper rate. Balanced and strong agni is fundamental to sound health.

It is extremely easy for the digestive fire to become imbalanced in pregnancy, while women are digesting for two. The digestive organs become compromised as pregnancy progresses and the baby grows, which shrinks the space and puts pressure on the intestines, stomach, and rectum. Pregnant women are susceptible to other digestive imbalances from hormonal shifts that can decrease bowel activity and relax and soften smooth intestinal muscles. This can cause food and waste to move slower through your system and create constipation. Increased levels of progesterone relax the muscles in the esophagus and stomach walls, leaving the flap (lower esophageal sphincter) that separates them slightly open, which makes it easier for stomach acid to travel up the esophagus. This creates an uncomfortable burning sensation, also known as acid reflux or heartburn.

Sometimes pregnant woman have such intense hunger that they can easily overeat, which can burden the stomach and digestive tract. It is often better to eat several small meals throughout the day instead of two or three large ones.

Incorporating dosha-appropriate spices into your cooking can kindle the digestive fire. Using spices *in normal amounts* is generally considered safe in pregnancy. All spices, including cinnamon, cloves, basil, oregano, ginger, cardamom, thyme, and rosemary, are generally good for Vata and Kapha types. Pitta types have the most restrictions, and benefit from cooling spices such as cilantro (coriander), fennel, mint, and dill. See the food charts in appendix 2 for a complete list of dosha-appropriate spices.

Carole was a Vata Pitta type and was experiencing Pitta imbalances in her pregnancy. Heartburn crept up on her in the afternoons and evenings after eating. She found simply using mint alleviated it tremendously. She

Kitchari

When you are having digestive troubles and want to give your system a break without depriving yourself of nutrients, eat kitchari, a dish at the core of Ayurvedic healing. It is a simple stew made from basmati rice and split mung beans with spices. There are endless variations of spices and vegetables you can add. Here is a tridoshic recipe.

Serves 4

Ingredients

1 cup basmati rice

½ cup yellow split mung beans (*not* yellow split peas)

3 tablespoons ghee

1 teaspoon fresh ginger, grated

1 pinch asafoetida (*hing*)

1 teaspoon black mustard seeds

1 teaspoon cumin seeds

½ teaspoon turmeric

1 (6-inch) piece of kombu, an edible type of kelp, high in minerals, that helps to soften beans while cooking, making them more digestible. (Available from natural food stores.)

4 cups water

½ teaspoon salt

1 handful cilantro, washed and chopped

(continued on the next page)

experimented with all forms of mint, including a couple of spoonfuls of mint ice cream, which worked very well!

JOURNALING EXERCISE

Observing How Food Affects Your Body

Observing how well you digest or don't digest your food, and food's effects on your energy/vitality and mood, can bring a new awareness to your diet that can help you make better choices to support your health. For three days:

- write down everything you consume—meals, beverages, and snacks—and what times of day you're eating;
- note if you were under stress or in a bad mood while eating.

In your diet diary, also write down your discoveries relative to your digestion, energy level, and mood. The following questions will help you to take a deeper look.

DIGESTION

- Observe how your belly feels; is there a sense of lightness and comfort, or heaviness and discomfort?
- Do you notice the presence or absence of gas and bloating?
- What is your breath like? Is there a pleasant or unpleasant smell and taste in your mouth?
- Did you have a bowel movement today? For example, maybe you have not had one in three days or maybe you had five before noon.

ENERGY LEVEL

- Does your energy feel balanced and stable? Or do you notice yourself feeling very tired and lethargic after eating certain foods or quantities of food?
- How does your energy level shift throughout the day relative to your eating?

MOOD

After eating do you feel:

- happy and light?
- irritable and angry?
- heavy and depressed? 🌢

General Guidelines for Improving Digestion

To truly nourish yourself with food, look beyond food lists and dos and don'ts. Examine how you eat and create healthy patterns for your mind and body. The following suggestions can help you get started. Try a few suggestions and notice how you feel. Attempt a few more and notice again. Strive not to become overwhelmed or discouraged as you slowly incorporate these guidelines into your life:

- Wash your hands before eating.
- Give thanks before each meal.
- Sip small amounts of warm water with meals and throughout the day. Don't drink a large glass of liquid with your meals.
- Eat in pleasant company with family or friends, or alone in silence. Try to avoid watching TV, reading the newspaper, or doing other activities while you eat so you can remain mindful while eating.
- Chew your food well, and bring your awareness to the tastes, smells, sounds, and textures of your food.
- Never overeat.
- Eat locally grown, fresh, seasonal foods, as much as possible.
- Eat foods whose qualities agree with you.
- Try to eat at regular meal times.

Directions

Make sure there are no stones in the mung. Soak for a few hours or overnight, then drain.

Wash rice and mung together, twice, and then drain.

In a medium-sized pot, heat ghee on medium heat until melted; add ginger, asafoetida, mustard, and cumin seeds. Sauté until mustard seeds begin to pop, then add turmeric, stirring quickly, and immediately add the rice/mung mixture. Stir for about 1 minute until the rice/mung mixture is well coated.

Add 4 cups of water and the kombu to the pot; stir and bring to a boil. Then lower the heat to medium, cover, and simmer for about 30 to 45 minutes until done. The kitchari should be very soft, but not gummy.

Add salt, stir, and serve, topped with fresh cilantro. On the side, enjoy with steamed or sautéed veggies, and chapattis/tortillas cooked in a cast-iron pan with ghee.

- Eat at home as much as possible, since the food you make at home holds the most loving energy and intentions.
- Avoid eating when you're upset, angry, bored, or depressed.
- Avoid sleep, intense study, exercise, and sex for at least two hours after eating.

Preparing the Kitchen

Now is the time to have fun in your kitchen! It feels great to cook in a clean, orderly environment. Remove clutter by discarding old kitchenware that you don't use, scratched pots and pans, and anything else creating disarray in your kitchen. This makes room for functioning cookware and utensils, and gives you space to feel comfortable attempting new recipes. Have a number of wooden spoons and spatulas, measuring cups and spoons, and cast-iron, stainless-steel, or glass pots and pans. Small hand graters for fresh ginger, cinnamon, nutmeg, and cheeses are helpful, as are metal strainers for rinsing grains and beans.

Cooking is an art and a wholesome activity that connects you to the natural world that gives us this bounty. Let wellness, wholeness, and inspiration guide your cooking endeavors. Stock your pantry with whole grains, dried beans, good-quality oils, unrefined sea salt, and fresh spices. Store grains, beans, and spices in glass jars behind cabinet doors to protect them from the heat of the sun and stove. Enliven your kitchen with abundant fresh produce, some fresh herbs, and dairy products (if you tolerate them well). Have bowls full of fresh fruit for you to snack on throughout the day, and keep plenty of healthy snacks available. Your kitchen and pantry will become beautiful and inspiring.

Remember the foods to favor and avoid when planning your meals. Try to make your meals as colorful as possible and pleasing to the eyes and senses. Not only will this stimulate the appetite, but it will also increase the enthusiasm of your family and friends when you are trying new foods and recipes. Thoroughly clean your kitchen when you're finished cooking. This will invite you back into your new domain to nourish yourself and your family.

Vegetarianism or Not?

Being a vegetarian is a very personal matter. There are a multitude of beneficial reasons to not eat meat. Some people choose to be vegetarian to promote nonviolence in general, and non-harming of animals specifically, while others choose it for health reasons (such as to lower cholesterol).

Some go vegetarian for its more sensible approach to caring for the environment and natural resources.

One misconception about Ayurveda is its stance on vegetarianism. Ayurveda does not implicitly state that you need to be a vegetarian. A vegetarian diet is considered desirable because it is sattvic and stands by the premise of *ahimsa*, or non-harming, but it is not required or necessarily appropriate for everyone.

There are some circumstances when eating meat is suggested. Pregnancy is one of these times. But there is controversy even among the classical texts. Some references advise the use of meat soups in pregnancy from the fourth month on, so a woman can keep up with her body's requirements for more protein, which supports the fetus's muscular-tissue growth. Other texts do not promote it.

If you do choose to eat meat, go for meat that is organic, local, and sourced from free-range and grass-fed animals. Prepare meat in soups or stews with ginger, turmeric, and other digestion-enhancing spices.

However, eating meat is *not* the only way to consume extra protein. You can be 100-percent vegetarian and experience excellent health in your pregnancy from a well-crafted diet. Vegetarian sources of protein include bean soups, stews, dips and burritos, tempeh, tofu, seitan, cottage cheese, yogurt, quinoa, nuts, seeds (and nut or seed butters), and shakes from rice, hemp, or whey protein.

Honoring Your Roots

Some women feel deeply connected to their ancestral roots. I have found that unearthing family food traditions can bring a deep sense of wellness and connection to your cultural history. I often encourage my clients to take a look at their families' culinary traditions and try to incorporate aspects of those traditions into their lives in a way that is appropriate for them. There may be situations when you are appalled by your traditional family foods, but if you are able to dig a little deeper, you may be surprised and find a few morsels to nibble on.

Isabella came to see me for digestive problems, including indigestion, gas, and bloating. She began to improve after adding herbal digestive support and restructuring her diet. But there was a missing piece to her puzzle that prevented total wellness. After our third session together, we discussed some of the underlying issues related to her digestive problems and what her diet was like growing up. She was from Colombia, and her mother frequently made slow-cooked chicken soup with heaps of fresh cilantro and corn. She revisited her family recipe, and one batch settled her stomach like no supplement could. Isabella decided to add more of her traditional foods into her diet to maintain and sustain her health.

Pregnancy is also an opportune time to ponder what cooking traditions you want to pass on to your children to give them culinary and cultural roots. Every time I cook lentil soup, I think of my grandfather growing lentils in a small village in Lithuania. I feel connected to a staple food that has brought strength and long life to my family for generations. Lentil soup was an essential fare in my pregnancies (also an incredible power-house of nutrients—protein, fiber, and iron, especially) and now my fresh pots of lentil soup are devoured completely by everyone in my family.

Honoring your ancestry through traditional foods is another step toward wholeness. Integrating the old with the new, ancient with modern, creates a bridge from the past to the present for you and your family. Hopefully you will enjoy your new creations of old family favorites, and feel connected to the strength in your relations, bringing more depth and richness to your life.

Vital Nutrients

No matter what your dosha, calcium, iron, protein, and essential fatty acids are vital nutrients in pregnancy.

CALCIUM

Calcium is necessary for the formation of the baby's bones and teeth, which begin to form as early as six to eight weeks in utero. Calcium is also extremely important in the last three months of pregnancy, when fetal bone formation makes significant strides. It is the most plentiful mineral in the body, and is essential for sustaining health in your bones, teeth, and connective tissue. Calcium also helps to nourish your nervous system, heartbeat, metabolism, and mineral balance throughout your body. Your baby will take the calcium he needs for his development, no matter how you eat or what you have stored. If you do not have adequate levels, you can easily become depleted. By focusing on calcium intake, it is easy to prevent imbalances like irritability, insomnia, leg cramps, cavities, and future bone loss.

The recommended dietary allowance (RDA) is 1000 mg to 1300 mg (not to exceed 2500 mg) of calcium daily in pregnancy. Calcium-rich foods include dark leafy greens (such as kale, spinach, and collards), yogurt, milk, cottage cheese and other cheeses, sesame seeds, sardines, salmon, tofu, and almonds.

IRON

Iron's main function is to combine with other nutrients to build the blood and form hemoglobin, the protein in red blood cells that carries oxygen to other cells. Iron aids protein metabolism, increases resistance to stress and diseases, and assists with proper muscle contraction. During pregnancy, the amount of blood in your body increases by 50 percent, so you need more iron to make more hemoglobin. You also need extra iron for your growing baby and placenta, especially in the second and third trimesters when you are building iron stores to transfer to your baby at birth, and for the first few months postpartum when you need to replenish your own red blood supply. Adequate iron intake can also prevent anemia caused by hemorrhaging during and after birth. (See appendix 1, "Remedies for Common Pregnancy Ailments," for more ideas on treating anemia. The RDA for iron is 27 milligrams per day for pregnant women.)

If you choose to supplement, avoid taking iron with a prenatal vitamin that contains calcium and magnesium, which inhibit iron's absorption. Be aware that many iron supplements can create constipation. On the other hand, many iron-rich foods, such as dried apricots and prunes, can have a laxative effect. You can increase your absorption of iron by cooking in cast-iron cookware and/or adding something acidic, such as lemon juice, to foods. When coffee and tea are consumed with food, it can greatly inhibit iron absorption.

Some disorders can arise from too much iron as well, so it is important to consume this mineral according to the recommended daily allowances. Iron-rich foods include edamame, lentils, chickpeas, pumpkin seeds, blackstrap molasses, tofu, dark leafy greens (such as kale, spinach, and collards), dry fruit (raisins, apricots, cherries), and animal protein (beef, turkey, chicken, and fish).

PROTEIN

According to Western science, protein is the building block that all bodily tissues rely on for growth. Protein comprises the uterus, placenta, skin, blood, muscles, bones, hair, nails, and all connective tissues. Protein also makes the soft and hard tissues that create your baby's body, and assists with your baby's hormones, growth, metabolism, and sexual development. This nutrient is extremely important in the production of brain cells. Blood sugar levels can stabilize from an adequate protein and carbohydrate ratio. Since protein is not well stored in the body, a steady supply is necessary. Many sources recommend 70 grams of protein a day in pregnancy. However, you can aim for that amount as an average over the course of a few days or a week. See page 51 for vegetarian sources of protein. Omnivores can receive their protein from eggs, chicken, fish, and other meats.

ESSENTIAL FATTY ACIDS (EFAS)

Essential fatty acids are lipids that cannot be synthesized within your body and must be ingested through your diet or from supplements. There are two families of EFAs, omega-3 and omega-6, and both are needed for physiologic functions including oxygen transport, energy storage, cell membrane function, and regulation of inflammation and cell proliferation.

American diets tend to be higher in omega-6s and too low in omega-3s. The most biologically active omega-3 fatty acids are eicosapentaenoic acid (EPA) and docosahexaenoic acid (DHA). Omega-3s are vital for optimal brain and retinal development in the fetus, and have demonstrated improved neurodevelopmental outcomes in children. Animal studies have shown that lack of omega-3 fatty acids during pregnancy is associated with visual and behavioral deficiencies that can't be reversed with postnatal supplementation. Omega-3 fatty acids may also play a role in preventing perinatal depression and reduction of asthma and other allergic conditions. It is best to supply these nutrients to the fetus throughout pregnancy.

Foods high in omega-3s include walnuts, pumpkin and flax seeds and their oils, DHA-enriched eggs, soybeans, tofu, seafood and fish (the FDA and EPA recommend limiting fish consumption to approximately twelve ounces of seafood per week *and* consuming fish and seafood with low levels of mercury; for example salmon, anchovies, and halibut). You may also choose to supplement with Prenatal DHA or Algae Omega (vegetarian DHA) from Nordic Naturals (see resources section) or another clean source, which I think is wise.

Sample Pregnancy Meals According to Body Type

The chart "Sample Meals by Dosha" contains ideas for pregnancy meals and snacks, and shows how each body type can enjoy a wide variety of foods in a balanced way. These examples are a blend of the ancient "science of life" and modern science. Foods with the qualities discussed in the beginning of this chapter are incorporated, along with foods thought to build ojas and increase sattva.

Along with these guidelines, remember the importance of enjoying your food and adopting a sense of lightness in your attitude. I am a firm believer in "everything in moderation"—even chocolate! Consciousness about your food choices does not need to become a rigid restriction. Food shopping, cooking, and eating should be pleasurable, joyous experiences. No one should feel burdened or stressed out from following a food list. Try to understand the general principles as best you can, experiment (you are your own best teacher), and enjoy!

Sample Meals by Dosha

	VATA	PITTA	KAPHA	TRIDOSHIC
BREAKFAST	Coconut-almond oatmeal with milk* Puffed rice cereal with roasted walnuts and almond milk Spinach-leek frittata with basil and goat cheese* and whole grain bread or roasted sweet potatoes	Coconut-almond oatmeal with milk* Delectable granola* with coconut or almond milk Egg white omelet with broccoli	Barley cereal with apricots, ground flax seeds, and cinnamon Delectable granola* with warm, spiced soy or rice milk Hard-boiled eggs with rye toast and a small amount of ghee	Cream of rice cereal cooked with raisins, cardamom, and milk of choice
LUNCH/ DINNER	Squash, carrot, and ginger soup* with sweet sesame baked tofu* and jazzed-up quinoa* Avocado spread on warm whole grain bread with cup of red lentil dal* and roasted asparagus Seitan-carrot stew over udon noodles or brown basmati rice	Black or pinto bean burrito with rice, goat cheese, lettuce, and cilantro Nori rolls with avocado, cucumber, tofu, and burdock Broccoli-ginger and soba stir-fry* with gomasio* and protein of your choice (tofu, salmon, or chicken)*	Rice noodles with white beans, kale, garlic, and basil Vegetable barley soup or curried cauliflower soup, with hummus on multigrain crackers Broccoli-ginger and soba stir-fry* with gomasio* and protein of your choice (tofu, salmon, or chicken)*	Mung dal kitchari (see recipe in this chapter, page 48) Aduki beans with fresh ginger Basmati rice pilaf with asparagus Most one-pot meals: since everything cooks for a long time, all the ingredients harmoniously blend together for all body types

Sample Meals by Dosha, continued

	VATA	PITTA	KAPHA	TRIDOSHIC
SNACKS	Tamari roasted walnuts, cashews, and almonds Seasonal fresh fruit (e.g., bananas, red grapes, or oranges) Soft, spreadable cheese on whole wheat chapatti	Roasted sunflower and pumpkin seeds Seasonal fresh fruit (e.g., pears, berries, dates) Cottage cheese	Dry roasted pumpkin and sunflower seeds Seasonal fresh fruit (e.g., berries, apples, pears, cherries) Lassi (yogurt blended with water) with cardamom	Fruit of choice Warm, gingered milk
BEVERAGES	Hot, gingered milk (whole milk or almond), plain or with blackstrap molasses Fresh squeezed orange juice Fresh pressed carrot, beet, and ginger juice	Hot, gingered (fresh) milk (1 or 2%) Pomegranate juice (preferably fresh) Fresh pressed celery, apple, kale, and carrot juice	Warm, spiced goat milk Apple juice or apple cider (preferably fresh) Fresh pressed carrot, beet, celery, and ginger juice	Nourishing pregnancy tea (see recipe in chapter 4, page 66) Fresh ginger tea

* Recipe included in appendix 3

Harmonious Lifestyle

A pregnant woman should be treated very attentively, as if (carrying) a vessel filled with oil (and trying) not to agitate.
Charaka Samhita, volume 1, chapter VIII

Peaceful Mother, Peaceful Baby

The intention for each and every day of your pregnancy is for a peaceful mother and a peaceful baby. *Charaka Samhita*, an ancient Ayurvedic text, tells us to treat a mother-to-be with gentle attention and care. It is said that whatever a mother takes in, including thoughts, emotions, experiences, and foods, both positive and negative, the baby becomes. Therefore, it is best to create as supportive a prenatal environment as possible.

Without putting undue pressure on yourself, begin to shift your thinking and activities to reflect the new journey you are embarking upon once your pregnancy is confirmed. One prominent Ayurvedic doctor believes that after conception takes place, the responsibility of creating happiness falls 80 percent on the woman. The remaining 20 percent falls on the partner, whose primary role is to create joy and support for the woman.

A simple place to begin the process of creating more peacefulness is your immediate surroundings. Fill your home with lots of light, healthy plants, and uplifting aromas, while cultivating cleanliness and order as much as possible. Do what you can to enhance an atmosphere of serenity in your work environment. You may enjoy pictures of places that bring happiness to you and the people you love, a small fountain that will allow you to hear the continuous peaceful sound of water, or an aromatherapy diffuser. Of course, there are many circumstances that can hinder a peaceful environment, such as toddlers who leave their trails of toys, clothing, and dirt throughout your home, or deadlines at work that create stress and chaos in your workspace. Try to remain "light" about these situations while doing what you can to maintain harmony around you.

To promote health and balance in our lives, we need a predominance of sattva. Sattva represents qualities that are positive and healthy, such as clarity, peacefulness, higher awareness, and intelligence. Striving for a sattvic lifestyle will positively influence the baby and its experience in the womb.

How can we experience more sattva within ourselves and in our relationships? Simple practices such as promoting positive thoughts and actions, being gentle and forgiving of yourself and others, going out of your way to make others feel better, always speaking the truth with kindness and compassion, and maintaining personal integrity will help. Creating time for spiritual practices, especially chanting and meditation, is important. Other sattvic activities include listening to peaceful music, singing, or reading uplifting books; eating pure, wholesome, and fresh foods; spending time in nature; and anything else healthy that delights your heart and soul.

It is a good idea to bathe daily and wear clean clothing. You may not want to spend a fortune on a new maternity wardrobe, but it is important to have clothes that feel and look good to you. White is often recommended because it is considered pure and able to hold the qualities of sattva. Other shades of colors that are soft, harmonious, and mild are beneficial as well. Gold jewelry is purported to make the uterus healthy, stabilize the fetus, and facilitate an easy delivery.

EXERCISE

Increasing Sattva in Your life

Begin to think of ways to feel more sattvic in your life:

- Are there practices and things you enjoy doing that create sattvic feelings?

- In the next week, try three new ideas to increase sattva. Try to be conscious of these actions as you move about your week.
- Do you notice a difference in your overall happiness, level of clarity, or anything else?

Since all of your experiences filter down to your baby, it is a good idea to avoid exposing yourself to images or sounds that are violent or upsetting, as they can create fear in the heart of your baby. These include disturbing movies and television programs, reading or hearing distressing stories, and listening to music that conjures up negative or hurtful imaginings. According to traditional Ayurvedic texts, visiting empty houses and cemeteries should be avoided during pregnancy, because they can create feelings of unsettledness.

While it's not possible to protect yourself completely from the stresses of life, difficult situations, or troubling encounters, you can let these experiences be opportunities to be gentle with yourself. Allow yourself time and space to process your emotions in whatever way works for you. If you talk to your baby and let her know what you're experiencing, she will be reassured by your calm voice.

As your hormones constantly surge during pregnancy, it is natural to feel a range of emotions within a single day. Ride the highs and let the joy and exuberance carry through in all that you do.

Pregnant women often emit a radiant glow, which is characteristic of the positive changes happening within. At the same time, they are extremely sensitive and become upset easily. The following ideas can help you to steady emotions in pregnancy:

- Pay extra attention to your diet to ensure an adequate intake of calories and regular, frequent meals and snacks. Make sure to eat enough protein, whole grains, healthy fats, fresh fruits, and vegetables.
- Perform daily self-care practices. (See "Healthy Daily Rhythms" later in this chapter, page 61.)
- Exercise, especially in fresh air, but any way you can. Find exercise that you enjoy and that is safe to do in pregnancy.
- Tune into your breath and bring awareness to the state of your mind and body. Practice yoga and breathing exercises appropriately.
- Write uncensored and freely in a journal. Express every troubling thought or upsetting emotion.

- Chant or sing. These can help to balance emotions by calming the heart and steadying the mind. (See the following section, "The Positive Use of Sound.")
- Create a support system for yourself. Stay connected to friends and family during your pregnancy, thus creating a network of people you feel safe and secure talking to about anything you are experiencing.

The Positive Use of Sound

Singing and chanting are uplifting and healing practices, especially when you recite sacred phrases. Vocalizing divine sounds, with meanings that resonate with your intentions, helps bring their meaning to life and their gifts to you.

These practices may also help to access parts of yourself previously unknown to you. In India, chanting was and is used as a tool for self-observation. While you are chanting or singing, you can hear the strength or weakness in your voice, you can notice if your mind is focused or distracted, and you can observe how you feel before and after.

In this book, I call chanting or singing exercises "sound practices." I chose to use chants in Sanskrit because of their connection to yoga and Indian sciences. The ones I have selected are universal in meaning, positive, and healing. They are not connected to any religion. However, if you would prefer to do a meaningful sound practice in another language or one connected to your spirituality or religion, please do so. The most important aspect is to provide a sacred vibration and positive energy for you and your baby.

In her first few months of pregnancy, Malia experienced a rough case of nausea that completely consumed all aspects her life. One of the few things she could do was sing. She used a fourth-century devotional Catholic chant to Mary to help her through this challenging time. Malia had heard the song once and it deeply resonated with her. She sang or lightly hummed the song every day to help move the energy of her morning sickness. Singing softly and gently created a lot of peace in her body, mind, and spirit. It became an opportunity for her to connect within and go to a silent place to be with her amazing miracle. She ended up singing the song every day for the rest of her pregnancy.

Using sound does not necessarily need to be a designated practice. Singing joyful sounds while you are cooking, bathing, doing daily chores, or taking a walk will still raise your spirits and foster contentment.

In my pregnancies, I loved singing while walking on the rural dirt roads of my neighborhood. Breathing in fresh air while I moved my body infused the songs with more life and got me out of my head. I recited Sanskrit mantras and sang Hebrew songs. Both helped me to feel connected to the source of life within me, and helped me absorb all the healing and uplifting vibrations from the sounds and nature. Afterward, I felt renewed every time.

As early as eighteen weeks into your pregnancy, the fetus can begin to hear. The baby's auditory development continues to progress as the network of nerves to the ears matures by twenty-eight weeks. At this point, the baby may recognize your and your partner's voices. While the validity of the Mozart effect (a theory that suggests listening to classical music can enhance intelligence) has come under close scrutiny, it has been proven that excessive noise can damage the fetus. Singing and chanting can be part of creating a nurturing and joyous sound environment that uplifts and soothes both you and your baby.

Chanting and sound in general, as powerful tools of expression, are very effective in helping women prepare for labor and in helping them give birth. When you use your voice in a positive way during labor, the sounds can help you feel rooted in your body and you can resist the temptation to tense up during contractions. Chanting helps to lengthen and deepen the breath and center the mind, which are other valuable preparations for labor.

There is a Zimbabwean proverb that says, "If you can walk, you can dance. If you can talk, you can sing." Even if you feel that you can't carry a tune—as many women do—you can still benefit from these practices by doing them in your authentic voice. Try to relax before and during the sound exercises in this book. Open your mouth wide and allow your voice to come forward. Let the sounds engage your heart, mind, breath, and body. You may also enjoy creating a ritual out of it or turning it into a meditation.

Healthy Daily Rhythms

Our everyday activities have a direct influence on our health. *Dinacharya* is the Sanskrit word for "daily routine." *Dina* means "day" and *charya* means "moving" or "following," so the phrase translates as "following the day."

Flowing with the natural rhythms and cycles of the sun, moon, and earth, and understanding their fluctuations bring us toward our healthiest, happiest, and most natural state. A daily routine is not meant to be a monotonous habit or rigid restriction, but an essential and enjoyable part of your life that brings a deeper sense of health. Dinacharya helps to keep stress at bay, maximize immunity, keep digestion strong, and increase resistance to disease.

In Ayurveda, great emphasis is placed on how your day begins because it sets the tone for what follows. Dinacharya follows the rhythms of the doshas that are naturally active at different times of the day. Vata governs the time between two and six o'clock (a.m. and p.m.), Pitta governs the time between ten and two o'clock (a.m. and p.m.), and Kapha governs the time between six and ten o'clock (a.m. and p.m.). Each of the general guidelines that follow is intended to balance the dosha most easily aggravated at that time of day.

All doshic types will want to follow these general guidelines, which can and *will* need to be modified for pregnancy and life with young children. (See the following sections.) These guidelines are meant to be just that: guidelines. You do not need to follow *every* recommendation; just find ones that work best for you. Change a few things at a time and notice how you feel, and then gradually incorporate what works into your daily rhythms. If changes are adopted slowly, over time their benefits will be sustained. After a while, these activities will become second nature as you move into a life of more harmony and balance. These Ayurvedic self-care rituals can encourage stability in body, mind, and spirit, especially when yoga, mantra, and meditation are emphasized.

GENERAL DAILY GUIDELINES FOR EVERYONE

- Wake with the sun.
- Go to the bathroom and empty your bladder and colon.
- Scrape your tongue, brush your teeth, and gargle with salt water.
- Rinse your nostrils with a neti pot.
- Drink a glass of room temperature or warm water.
- Do self-massage and bathe. (See "An Essential Practice: The Ayurvedic Self-Massage" in this chapter on page 68.)
- Perform some kind of spiritual practice (asana, pranayama, meditation, chanting, prayer) or physical exercise.
- Eat breakfast in a calm, relaxed setting.
- Work, study, or perform other responsibilities.
- Eat lunch in a calm, relaxed setting.

- Continue work or other duties from the morning.
- Perform some kind of spiritual practice (asana, pranayama, meditation, chanting, prayer) or exercise.
- Eat dinner in a calm, relaxed setting.
- Spend time with family or friends, relax, or read.
- Go to sleep before 10 p.m.

Daily Rhythms for Each Dosha

When you have an understanding of your doshic constitution, you can take steps every day to follow a lifestyle that is in harmony with both your innate nature and the natural world.

VATA

The main goals for Vata types are to maintain regular, consistent routines for meal times, sleep, and work, with plenty of time for resting and nourishing the body and mind. Vata types should create schedules that allow for some flexibility to ebb and flow with their erratic nature. It is important to leave time to rest as much as possible after intense periods of work, study, or other challenging endeavors. Vata types benefit from making every effort to stay warm and calm. They will want to eat three meals at regular times consisting of ample, warm, and moist foods. A hot breakfast is essential!

Vata rules the junctures of the day, sunrise and sunset, and the larger span of time between 2:00 and 6:00 a.m. and 2:00 and 6:00 p.m. During these times Vata tends to be the most active, which makes it easy to feel scattered, and creates susceptibility to imbalance. Vatas will often wake up during this time frame in the morning. These hours are wonderful for meditation, asana practice, chanting, and creativity, especially when you've slept sufficiently the night before. To promote adequate sleep, go to bed early (before 10:00 p.m.) after having had a warm milk drink, a warm bath, and sesame oil massaged onto the soles of the feet.

Between two and six in the afternoon, many people feel a dip in their energy. Vata types benefit from taking a short rest between two and four in the afternoon. They may want to use this time for quiet reflection or

Neti Pot Rinse

Neti pots are small vessels that look like Aladdin's lamp, and you fill them with pure water and sea salt to rinse and cleanse your nasal passages. They work wonders to alleviate congestion, sinus problems, allergies, headaches, and more, as they rinse away pollution, dust, pollen, and other irritants. They are safe to use in pregnancy and can be part of your morning and/or evening routine. Neti pot rinses are especially great after air travel. They are available from your local drugstore or from the Ayurvedic suppliers listed in the resources section at the end of the book.

Follow the instructions that are included with the pot, or you can even watch a video on youtube.com to see how it's done.

restorative breathing and yoga practices. If these are not possible, Vata types should try to minimize intense activities and schedules during this time. Taking natural and herbal energy boosts such as chyavanprash or a rejuvenating ojas drink (see chapter 3, page 43) can be beneficial in this window of time.

Moderate exercise, such as swimming and walking, is excellent for Vata types. Listening to peaceful music or to the sound of streams, rivers, oceans, or fountains nourishes Vata types' delicate nervous system. Colors should be soft, warming, and calming (the opposite qualities of Vata) rather than bold and bright. Gold, red, orange, and yellow (not bright) combined with white or whitish-blue and green are good colors for Vata. While black, gray, and brown may help ground Vata when necessary, too much can be depressing and devitalizing. Aromas such as lavender and sweet orange can be used to nourish Vata types as well, especially in times of aggravation. (Please see appendix 6 for how to use essential oils safely.)

PITTA

The primary intention for Pitta types is to practice moderation in all endeavors. They also need three regular meals of moderate quantity, favoring cooling and soothing foods. It is best to avoid hot, spicy, sour, and oily foods, and to limit salt intake. Ideally, Pittas should have sufficient challenges to keep them occupied without the stress and intensity of severe competition, even though they thrive on that.

Pitta governs the hours between 10:00 a.m. and 2:00 p.m., which are times of great alertness and productivity. Agni mirrors the movement of the sun, with its rays strongest around noon. This is the perfect time to eat your biggest meal of the day. Pitta also governs from 10:00 p.m. to 2:00 a.m. Falling asleep after 10:00 p.m. can increase the fiery Pitta energy, forming a "second wind" that leads to insomnia.

Excelling in sports is natural for Pitta types. However, they need to be careful with too much competition and drive, which can overpower them. Water-based sports are excellent. Pitta types should exercise during the coolest part of the day, and avoid exposure to excessive heat, steam, and sunshine.

Pitta types benefit from music and aromas that are sweet and soothing. Lavender and sandalwood are good essential oils. White, green, blue—even gray and other cool, mild, calming colors, preferably in pastel or other mild shades, are balancing colors for Pittas. They should avoid hot colors like red, orange, and yellow, as well as deep black.

KAPHA

The key aims for Kapha types are to stimulate and invigorate the body, mind, and senses. Kapha types need to vary their routine, get plenty of exercise, and stay active. They often do better eating two meals a day. Breakfast can be skipped (though not in pregnancy) or consist of fresh fruit or spiced tea. The diet should emphasize light, warm, dry foods with pungent spices, generally avoiding dairy products and other heavy foods. Hot, warm, or room-temperature drinks are best.

Kapha types benefit from setting goals and creating challenging situations to stay engaged. They must make a conscious effort to create variety in all their pursuits. They need zest. Competition is good for them, although they may find it stressful. Kaphas need to create heat, energy, and stimulation. They should not nap during the day, which can clog the bodily channels and create more lethargy and heaviness.

Kapha governs the hours between 6:00 and 10:00 a.m. and 6:00 and 10:00 p.m. Most Kapha types benefit from rising before Kapha is activated in the morning, otherwise a sense of heaviness can make it difficult to get moving. This is an excellent time of day for cleansings, evacuations, and ridding the body of excess Kapha accumulations, such as phlegm. A daily neti cleanse with warm, salted water can clear up Kapha congestion in the sinuses.

Vigorous exercise is wonderful for Kapha types if they can muster the motivation to get started. Tennis, jogging, dancing, and aerobics are some good choices. They should strive for daily exercise. Warm, stimulating, and bright colors like red, orange, gold, and yellow are good for Kaphas, as opposed to rich, dark colors that can aggravate them. If blue or green is used, the brighter hues should be favored. To spice things up, Kaphas can handle sharp contrasts in color. Invigorating, pungent, and uplifting aromas, such as grapefruit and eucalyptus, benefit Kapha.

Daily Rhythms in Pregnancy

If the concept of a daily rhythm or dinacharya is new to you, you may find pregnancy is a wonderful time to begin your self-care practices. The time you take to nurture yourself will benefit you and your baby immensely. Remember that all your activities should be gentle and easy. Now is not the time to try waking at four in the morning for pranayama (breathing practices). Ample sleep is essential in pregnancy and often difficult to achieve. Going to bed by ten, naturally waking at six, and then beginning your morning practices is a more sensible goal.

Mother's Nourishing Tea

An essential daily activity in pregnancy is savoring a mug of mineral-rich herbal tea. Nettle leaf is an herb loaded with many vitamins and minerals, most notably iron. Raspberry leaf is purported to strengthen the uterus, making the herb a great preparation for labor. Milky oats are food for your nervous system. Rosehips boost a little vitamin C, and the orange peel and peppermint add a pleasant flavor, digestive support, and harmonize the blend. Some women like mint and find that it helps with nausea, while others find that it aggravates their heartburn. Omit mint if it does not agree with you.

This tea is safe to drink throughout your pregnancy and postpartum time. See the resources section for where to purchase bulk herbs.

(continued on the next page)

Many of the guidelines set forth in previous sections can be done in pregnancy, except:

- Kapha types benefit from daily exercise but *not* vigorous exercise such as aerobics. Kapha types ought to use pungent spices in normal amounts and not skip breakfast. Make it a light breakfast or a small quantity if hunger isn't strong.
- Waking with the sun if you had trouble sleeping the night before.

Amira had been living an Ayurvedic lifestyle for years before becoming pregnant. After each of her pregnancies was confirmed, she shifted her dinacharya practice by adding special pregnancy-belly massage oil into her daily self-massage routine. Amira enjoyed going deeper in her meditation practice in her first pregnancy, but had difficulty finding time to continue meditating in her second pregnancy when she had a young child to take care of. She knew that she could return to meditating at some point in the future when her family life permitted more time for it.

Because the doshas are different, the daily routine for a Vata type will differ greatly from that of a Kapha type. For example, a pregnant Vata woman may require an afternoon nap. Her nervous system will be calmed and she can catch up on inadequate sleep from the previous night. But a pregnant Kapha woman may feel considerably heavier and lethargic after an afternoon nap, so napping is not advised for this type—unless the previous night was very short on sleep. Follow the guidelines for your predominant dosha.

Exercise is an essential aspect to emphasize in a daily routine during pregnancy. It can improve your mood, digestion, and energy level, and help with sound sleep, stress reduction, and relaxation. Regular exercise also keeps your weight gain reasonable, improves circulation, and builds the strength, stamina, and flexibility that you will need for labor and birth. Walking, hiking, swimming, and yoga are great for all body types. You may also enjoy using stationary bikes, elliptical trainers, and treadmills. It's best for Vata types to approach exercise in a gentle and soothing way, Pitta types in a relaxed and noncompetitive manner, and Kapha types with enthusiasm and consistency.

Daily Rhythms for Women with Babies and Young Children

When you have youngsters, your daily rhythm can easily fall by the wayside. If you need to wake during the night to feed your baby, sleeping in later in the morning may be essential. In the first few months of motherhood, you may feel there is barely enough time to take care of basic necessities like bathing, brushing your teeth, or preparing food. You may have a toddler who requires your help in the mornings, which can throw a wrench into your daybreak practices. Anyone with school-age children knows the morning busyness of preparing breakfast, school lunches, and getting the children ready for the day. The focus of those precious early hours previously devoted to self-care is replaced with caring for your family, unless you wake up quite early. But it all becomes easier once your children reach a certain age.

Do the best you can! Pick and choose the morning rituals that support you the most. Squeeze in what you can and *let go* of the rest. Do not berate yourself for not following all the guidelines you would like every day. Being a present, loving parent is most important. If you have a partner or someone else helping you care for your children, negotiate with them to help you carve out time on the weekends to take care of yourself.

Integrate your young children into your daily rhythms and encourage them to participate in their own way. This can help build a bridge between your self-care and caring for your family. When my daughter was three, she loved to do self-massage with me. (See the next section, "An Essential Practice: The Ayurvedic Self-Massage.") I would set out a big towel on the bathroom floor along with a jar of coconut oil. We had so much fun massaging ourselves, then jumping into the bath or shower together. Children are such tactile creatures and love to play with sticky, gooey substances. I

Ingredients
2 cups nettle leaf
2 cups raspberry leaf
2 cups milky oats (also called oat tops)
¼ cup rosehips
¼ cup orange peel
¼ cup peppermint leaf

Directions
Mix the herbs together in a large bowl, then store in a glass jar with a lid in a cool, dark place. Place a quarter of a cup of the mixed herbs in a quart of boiling water. Put a lid on it and steep for 30 to 90 minutes. Strain and sweeten with honey or apple juice, if desired. Drink it warm throughout the year and at room temperature or cool in the summer. Enjoy a few cups daily.

remember the first time we did this together; she could not believe we could play with creamy oil and rub it all over our bodies.

Children also learn by example. When they see how you care for yourself, they will naturally want to mirror you. My daughter loves to hear me chant, and sometimes we practice yoga together. While at times I prefer to do these rituals alone in a quiet space, it's not always possible. Sharing these practices has other benefits for both of us, including the sense of closeness it creates.

Little things like eating in calm, relaxed settings can be difficult with busy, young children. Light a candle and say a prayer of thanks, as a family, before your meal. This can at least help to set the tone for a peaceful mealtime.

Sunita has two young boys, ages five and nine, and finds that mealtime and bedtime rituals help her whole family. Everyone benefits from the regular, predictable routine. When her boys were younger, she put her meditation practice on hold. Now that her oldest son is nine, she meditates with him; he enjoys both the practice and the special time with his mom.

JOURNALING EXERCISE

Your Daily Rhythms

Take out your journal and write freely based on the following questions:

- Do you already have a daily rhythm—even a general one? If so, write it down. If not, how do you feel about the idea?
- Which practices would you like to try? Make a list of your ideal day with daily self-care practices. Make sure to include exercise you enjoy.
- Commit to trying out your ideal day for at least two weeks.
- After two weeks, observe how you feel with your new rhythm. In what ways is your overall day different? ◗

An Essential Practice: The Ayurvedic Self-Massage

One of the most fundamental self-care practices in pregnancy is the daily *gentle* oil massage. For thousands of years, people in India have used daily oil massage, called *abhyanga* (pronounced ah-be-an-ga), as a health-promoting ritual. Abhyanga is an excellent practice in all stages of life, but is especially important in pregnancy since the body goes through its own metamorphosis to accommodate the new life developing and growing inside the womb. The more you are in touch with your body and can support its changes, the easier and more comfortable you will feel, and the more resistance you will have to ward off imbalance and illness.

Of all the sense organs in the body, the skin is the largest, with more surface area and sensory receptors than any other organ. For this reason, when oil is massaged into the skin, circulation increases throughout the whole body. Abhyanga nourishes and strengthens the immune system by creating another layer of defense to protect the body from the constant bombardment of the external environment. This layer of defense can increase your resistance to disease and imbalance, while boosting your stamina.

Studies have shown that pregnant women who are massaged twice a week for a period of twenty minutes reported less anxiety, improved quality of sleep, improved mood, and less back pain. These women also had fewer complications in labor and fewer postnatal complications. If you have the means, you can hire a massage therapist on a regular basis. However, a similar effect can be achieved by frequent light self-massage (abhyanga) at home, which can also become a delightful ritual.

Snehana (pronounced snay-hana) is a Sanskrit word that means both "oiling" and "loving." Abhyanga is a type of snehana. The effects of abhyanga are believed to be similar to those we experience when we are bathed with love. This practice brings a deep sense of warmth and security, like the feeling of being loved. I have found this to be true, and many of my clients have discovered similar feelings from a regular routine of Ayurvedic self-massage. They reported fewer feelings of agitation, an increased sense of balance, more energy throughout the day, more calmness at night, and radiantly glowing skin.

The practice of abhyanga can take as little as five minutes during your daily routine. On busy days, you can skip the head, and massage only the body while you're in the shower. If you have more time, you can spend up to thirty minutes. The cumulative effects of abhyanga create a protective seal on the body and an energy field that is beneficial during pregnancy, a time when it is natural to feel more vulnerable. When you set aside time to connect and nurture yourself by doing abhyanga, your growing babe soaks up all that loving touch before it even enters the world!

HOW TO DO SELF-MASSAGE

You will need ¼ to ½ cup of oil and an old towel designated as your "oil towel." (The following section discusses the types of oil appropriate for your body type.) Your oil towel will get stained and eventually saturated with oil. After washing the towel with a little extra laundry soap, dry it on low heat in the dryer to avoid combustion from oily residue.

Pour oil into a small glass or plastic squeeze bottle, then place it in hot water for five minutes to warm the oil. Then sit or stand comfortably in a warm room on your oil towel. Make sure there are no cold drafts or wind. Alternatively, you can massage yourself while in the shower.

As everything in pregnancy should be soft and gentle, so too is the massage. No vigorous or deep massage! Begin by anointing the crown of your head with a small amount of oil and then massage your scalp in circles. Give some time to all parts of your ears, then massage your face in upward motions, from chin to ears and nose to ears. You will eventually lightly massage your entire body, using long, up-and-down strokes on the long bones of your arms and legs, and circular motions around your joints.

Lovingly massage your breasts from the periphery to the nipples to relieve any tenderness and to prepare for nursing. Spend extra time oiling your belly *very gently* in a large clockwise direction and letting your hands feel the pulse of your growing baby. Follow the large intestine by moving up the right side of your body, across the center, and down the left side. You may notice the belly needs more oil to alleviate itchiness or dryness that commonly results from the skin stretching. This is a nice time to connect with the little soul inside and to express joy and excitement for her arrival by communicating just that with your hands on your belly.

There are no definitive answers about why some women develop stretch marks and others do not. It may be related to heredity, tissue strength, elasticity of the skin, or nutrition. Abhyanga can help regardless of the cause. As pregnancy progresses and the baby becomes larger, abhyanga can help to alleviate upper and lower backache and sciatica if more time is spent on those trouble spots.

Continuing down, massage in large circular strokes around your hips, knees, and ankles, and up-and-down strokes on your legs. The perineum (the area of skin between your *yoni* and rectum) can also be gently massaged (from week thirty-four until delivery) to help prepare for labor and decrease the chances of tearing, especially for women who have not given birth before. The self-massage is not complete without massaging your feet. This relieves coarseness, stiffness, cracking soles, fatigue, and helps you sleep.

Ideal times for this practice are after waking up and before going to bed. When you are finished, you can jump into a warm shower or bath. Let the excess oil be rinsed away by warm water, not soap. You can use soap on just those spots that tend to harbor odor and bacteria. You may need to shampoo twice to rinse all the oil out of your hair, unless some oil in your hair doesn't bother you. Alternatively, you can massage yourself after bathing with a very light coat of oil and then put on clothes that you don't mind getting a little oily. The longer the oil stays on to soak in and nourish your skin, the better.

CHOOSING OILS

When choosing an oil to use for abhyanga, it is important to consider both your body type and the time of year. Vata types will want to use oils that have the qualities of warmth and heaviness, such as almond or sesame. Pittas want to control heat in the body and mind, and do well with cooler oils, such as sunflower and coconut. Kapha types do best with lighter oils, like sunflower, or warming oils (to improve circulation), such as sesame.

Most of us are dual types and can mix and match oils according to our current state of health and cycles of the year. For example, I am a Pitta Vata type. In the summer, when I tend to run hotter, I use coconut oil. In the winter when my skin is drier and I feel colder, I use sesame. Experiment to find the right oil for you.

After you discover which oil is best, you can make herbal oil by infusing herbs into the oil to enhance its therapeutic and nourishing effects. See appendix 5, "How to Make Herbal Oils," for instructions.

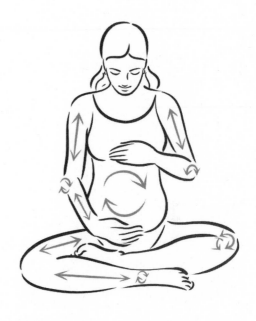

figure 1 **When massaging your body,** use long, up-and-down strokes on the long bones of your arms and legs, and circular motions around your joints and belly.

PART TWO

Your Pregnancy

A Month-by-Month Guide

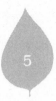

5

The First Trimester

Your own positive future begins in this moment. All you have is right now.
Every goal is possible from here.
LAO TZU

Welcome to *your* pregnancy! You've probably just taken a home
pregnancy test and are adjusting to the news. You may want to
announce your pregnancy to everyone under the sun, or perhaps keep the
news limited to a few trusted souls for now. Do what feels right for you.

The first three months of pregnancy are filled with immense change. To
help you adapt to all that pregnancy brings, set aside time every day or
several days a week for the practices outlined in this book. This will help
you feel as content, balanced, and relaxed as possible.

What follows in this chapter is a brief guide to the baby's development in the first trimester, with typical physical and emotional changes
you may experience. The second and third trimesters will be explored
in chapters 9 and 13, respectively. The information presented is based
on modern medicine, Ayurvedic teachings, and my own observations
and experience. It is important to remember that there are always variations within the normal range. Every woman's experience of pregnancy
is unique, whether it is her first or her fifth. Also, please keep in mind
that there is an immeasurable element of mystery during pregnancy that
continually creates new experiences.

What's Happening in Your Body?

The first trimester brims with growth and development. During this phase, the fetus's major organs and the central nervous system begin to develop. The face, eyes, ears, nose, toes, fingers, chin, lips, and mouth begin to form. The heart starts beating in the fourth week. Brain cells are growing rapidly. By the end of the seventh week, all the essential structures have been formed, both internally and externally. The baby can respond to touch and make gentle movements. By twelve weeks, the uterus is the size of a large grapefruit.

Since this is a highly developmental stage for the baby, avoid alcohol, drugs, and exposure to chemicals, cigarettes, and environmental toxins.

TYPICAL PHYSICAL CHANGES

Within two weeks of conception, hormones trigger your body to begin nourishing your baby. Many women begin to experience physiological changes as early as those first two weeks. You may notice:

- Tender breasts. The increase of hormones can make your breasts feel fuller, heavier, and more sensitive.
- Nausea and vomiting. Many women experience morning sickness or nausea and vomiting (NVP). As unpleasant as it is, NVP is a normal and healthy response to pregnancy.
- Fatigue. You may feel unusually tired in the first trimester as your body adjusts to the pregnancy.
- Frequent urination. You might find yourself urinating more often than usual, especially at night. Pressure on your bladder from the enlarging uterus can cause you to leak urine when coughing, laughing, or sneezing.
- Spotting. Some women experience light spotting or bleeding five to ten days after conception. This can be a sign that the embryo has implanted itself on the uterine wall. It is a normal, common condition. Contact your prenatal care provider if the bleeding persists or if you are concerned.

TYPICAL EMOTIONAL CHANGES

Adjusting to pregnancy is monumental and can add stress to your life, whether the baby is a planned or unplanned addition. It may take a few months to get used to the idea that you are pregnant. You may feel ecstatic, scared, or exhausted at different times, or all at once.

Some women find themselves confronting body-image issues as they gain weight, yet still do not look pregnant. Hormonal changes can create mood swings and emotional sensitivities. It may feel overwhelming to have nausea, fatigue, and intense hunger pangs on top of it all. These are all natural feelings and responses to pregnancy.

You may wonder how the new baby will affect your relationship with your partner or other children. Let this be an opportunity to openly communicate with your partner about your concerns. The baby may also influence your work and finances. Use this time to explore creative ideas relative to your job and financial situation, if these are relevant to you.

If you are embarking on pregnancy as a single woman, choose a close friend or two for special support in this chapter of your life. She or he can accompany you to your office visits or other classes typically attended by couples, and simply act as a supportive presence to and affirmation of your pregnancy.

Now is a good time to start a dialogue with yourself and partner or friend about what kind of prenatal care and birth you would like. There are many options today, and selecting your prenatal provider is a very personal decision. Whether you decide to use a midwife, obstetrician, or family practice doctor, it is most important that you trust your practitioner and that you resonate with her style of practice. Interview several healthcare providers, ask questions, and talk with other mothers in your community about their experiences. A new trend among some providers is to offer group prenatal appointments. This type of care brings together women in similar stages of pregnancy for their prenatal office visits. Usually there is an educational component that addresses some aspect of pregnancy, from prenatal nutrition to pain-coping strategies for labor, and there is always personal time with your provider to check your vitals.

My husband and I used a midwife for our first child because we wanted to birth at home. We savored every hour-long prenatal visit in our midwife's home office, asking questions, learning about my body and the pregnancy, getting to know each other and building a good, positive relationship. We chose group prenatal care in a women-centered practice for my second pregnancy. The group prenatal care created a wonderful bonding experience with other pregnant women, and I still meet with many of the mothers now as we watch our little ones grow up together. Both were enriching, educational, and enjoyable experiences.

6

Month One

INTUITION AND DREAMING

The intuitive mind is a sacred gift and the rational mind is a faithful servant.
We have created a society that honors the servant and has forgotten the gift.
ALBERT EINSTEIN

Intuition is the product of persistent perception," Dr. Vasant Lad non-chalantly said in one of his lectures at the Ayurvedic Institute years ago. I paused, pondered for a moment, and jotted his idea down in my note-book, knowing that at some point I would contemplate it further.

I hadn't returned to his statement until I began writing this book, and could not help but think about the importance of building intuition early in pregnancy, and using it as a tool now and throughout motherhood. Intuition can help you navigate through the seasons of your pregnancy, and later, your family life, as you make choices for the small beings under your wing. When life throws you challenges that you cannot sort out with the logical mind, intuition can be a great support and tool to provide guid-ance, understanding, and clarity.

Intuition is an instinctive knowledge or belief that is independent of any reasoning process. Is it a mysterious force or a highly specialized way of thinking? Perhaps both. Have you ever taken a different route home for some unknown reason and avoided an accident? Do you get a feeling in your gut when confronted with a difficult decision about what you *know* you should do? These examples are intuition in action.

Women are inherently intuitive, but this skill can be enhanced through increased and continuous awareness or perception, as Dr. Lad indicated. When you observe yourself—your feelings, thoughts, actions, and reactions to the world around you—you create more consciousness and understanding. Yoga philosophy presents the idea of *svadhyaya*, self-observation or self-inquiry, as a tool for self-growth and a step toward creating positive changes in your life. Self-observation and contemplation help you tune into the part of yourself that naturally knows what to do. Your intuition may tell you to do something that you do not understand, but trusting it allows you to believe in your insights.

Pregnancy is a time of heightened awareness and unusually keen sense perception, which makes it an opportune time to harness inner wisdom and develop intuition. The process begins with pausing. Having a baby is a major life transition, and pausing allows you to stop, pay attention, and move through this transition from your inner place of knowing. Your intuition is always accessible if you know how to tune into it. How can you cultivate intuition?

- Take quiet time every day and set an intention to receive the information you need.
- Listen to the cues in your body, especially your stomach/gut and heart.
- Open your mind to the information that comes, whatever it may be.

Dreams

Your inner journey to deeper self-awareness and enhanced mental and physical well-being during pregnancy can include learning from your dreams. Messages, spoken and unspoken, are revealed through the dream world, illuminating what is not in your present conscious state of awareness. Sometimes you can process emotions or situations through your dreams that you cannot in your day-to-day life. Recurring patterns, unresolved issues, and a deeper self-understanding are revealed through attention to dreams.

Ayurveda views dreams as connected to the *majja dhatu,* one of the seven tissues of the body; it is the tissue related to the nervous system and bone marrow. This idea supports the belief that dreams are connected with nervous discharges related to mental impressions acquired throughout the day. Ayurveda sees this connection as a natural way to bring closure to unfinished thoughts, emotions, and actions.

The underlying causes of imbalance and disease can be understood through dreams, which begin the process of mental, emotional, and physical healing. Ayurveda views illnesses as stemming from imbalances in the mind. By understanding the movement of thought patterns in dreams, you can understand an imbalance more clearly. Recognizing the influence of the doshas on dreams sheds light into the nature of your dream. Then you can take steps to balance the dosha and eventually heal the problem. All dreams are classified as Vata, Pitta, or Kapha, each presenting particular characteristics.

Vata dreams are usually very active, with movements such as running, flying, jumping, and falling. They also include anxiety, fear, panic, confusion, and being pursued, frozen, or dead.

Pitta dreams often entail intensity, passion, problem-solving, teaching, and studying. Pitta types of emotions usually appear, including anger; criticism/judgments; aspects of fire, such as a house burning; arriving somewhere late; failing; and being naked in public.

Kapha dreams include romance, desires, sentimentality, and watery representations. Kapha emotions include attachment, lethargy, and slowness. Swimming, snow, lakes, and rivers also appear in Kapha dreams.

You may not be aware of how a dosha is particularly imbalanced until its message comes to you in a dream. One summer I began to feel heat rise in my system while I was working on the deadline for this book. I started feeling a little sharp with my children, but wasn't completely aware how much Pitta was accumulating in me until I had a dream that the house where I lived in college burned down. When I reflected on the intensity of the dream, the heat, fire, and burned-down house, it made me realize that Pitta had become quite aggravated. The dream showed me that I needed to take steps to pacify Pitta, *before* it became provoked even more. I made a conscious effort to follow a Pitta-pacifying diet, and made a point not to be outside in the heat of the day, unless by the side of a pool or ocean, sipping coconut water. Eventually the heat in my system lessened. I was thankful for the insight the dream had revealed.

Sweet Dreams Mama

Warm, spiced milk before bed brings relaxation and induces sound sleep. Warm 1 cup of the milk of your choice, add a pinch of cardamom and turmeric (suggested to give your baby beautiful skin) and drizzle in honey or maple syrup.

Sandalwood essential oil is purported to promote tranquility, enhance deep sleep, and create a vivid dream state. Place a diffuser with sandalwood oil in your bedroom or rub a drop onto your palms and then on your pillowcase.

Warm sesame oil massaged onto the soles of your feet promotes sound sleep. You may want to put socks on afterward to prevent oil stains on your sheets.

Herbal pillows or sachets are small pillows filled with calming, fragrant herbs that induce sound sleep and promote peaceful dreams. They can be placed inside your larger pillow or in your bed. Buy one filled with dried lavender flowers at your local farmers market or make your own in the shape of a moon or heart or rectangle.

In appendix 1, "Remedies for Common Pregnancy Ailments," under "Insomnia," there are more tips on achieving a restful slumber and sweet dreams.

JOURNALING EXERCISE

Dream Journal

A dream journal is a special diary in which to record your dreams and the reflections and feelings evoked by them. Writing down your dreams helps you remember them and preserve the details, which would otherwise be rapidly forgotten no matter how significant the dream seemed. The practice of recording dreams can also help to improve future dream memory. Look at this activity as an interesting and fun way to gain insight into your inner soul. There is no right or wrong way to keep a dream journal, but here are a few ideas to get started:

- Commit to writing in a dream journal for at least two weeks.
- Place your journal and pen, colored pencils, or markers next to your bed for easy access.
- Before you go to bed, remind yourself that you will be journaling in the morning and looking for insights. Write tomorrow's date in your journal so you do not have to think about it when you wake up.
- In the morning, write down everything you remember as soon as you wake up. Try to include colors, feelings, textures, actions, and shapes to describe your experiences. If you have time and feel inclined, add some drawings of images you remember. Don't worry if you don't remember many details at first.

If you have time in the morning, also write down your thoughts about your dream and any associations you can think of, or return to your journal later in the day when you have more time. Ask yourself:

- What was revealed to you?
- Do you see a connection to the characteristics of the doshas? Which one(s)?
- Do you need to do anything differently to bring balance to your life? 💧

BREATHING PRACTICE

Relaxing and Calming the Breath

Sukhasana, or easy pose, is a base pose for this and many more of the breathing and meditation practices that you will be doing throughout all trimesters.

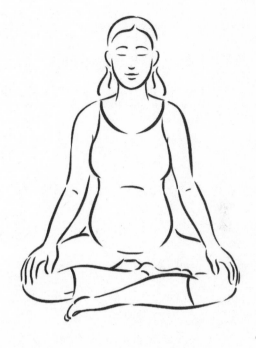

- Sit on your buttocks on the floor. You may wish to use a blanket to elevate your hips for increased comfort. If you use a blanket, choose a thick one and fold in half so it is about two to six inches high. Then sit on your buttocks on the blanket.
- Widen your legs, and bend your knees so that you can slip each foot beneath the opposite knee as you fold your legs in toward your torso.
- Make sure the pelvis is in a neutral position, neither tilted forward nor backward.
- Take a deep breath and feel your spine lengthen as you sit tall and relax your feet, legs, shoulders, and arms.
- Rest your hands on your thighs.

figure 2 **Sukhasana**

Now that you are comfortable in Sukhasana, or just sitting cross-legged or in a chair, we will move into the breathing practice.

With this practice, you will explore gentle breath awareness, then bring your attention to extended exhale breathing, which has a calming and relaxing effect on your mind and body. Extended exhale breathing can be done before bed, if you awake in the middle of the night, or any time you feel agitated and wish to become more tranquil.

Pranayama exercises are typically done in a seated position, but in pregnancy, your comfort is paramount and *all pregnant women can bend the rules as needed.*

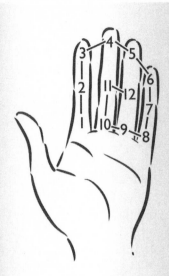

figure 3 **Counting Your Breaths**

Counting Your Breaths

A simple way to keep track of your repetitions while doing breathing practices is to count on the inner digits of your hand. Begin by placing your thumb at the base of your index finger (number one) on the inside of your hand. After each complete breath, to remind you of your place, move your thumb to the next numbered position (see Figure 3). Keep moving in a spiral until you have touched all of your digits and reached a count of twelve. This counting method is based on an old Indian ritual to facilitate twelve repetitions of one type of pranayama.

If you are feeling especially tired, you may prefer to do this exercise lying down. If you are in the first trimester, you can rest on your back with your knees bent and feet flat on the floor. If you are returning to this exercise later in your pregnancy, in the second and third trimesters, you can lie on your side, supported by pillows under your head and between your legs.

- Keep your eyes closed for this practice. Breathe through your nose, with your mouth closed. Throughout the practice, keep a gentle smile on your face.
- Place your palms on your belly and bring your awareness to your breathing.
- Breathe naturally for a few moments. With each inhalation and each exhalation, feel your hands as your belly moves them.
- Now take a few slower breaths, still feeling the subtle movements of your belly rising and falling. Let each breath be full and complete.
- Continue to breathe naturally as you inhale. But then, use just a little effort to encourage all your breath to leave as you exhale.
- Inhale naturally, feeling your body's expansion, and then gently and gradually, without too much effort, make your exhales a little longer and fuller.
- Continue to progressively deepen your breath. Be gentle. Inhale naturally, feeling your body's expansion. Gently and gradually make your exhale a little longer and fuller, but without too much effort. After a few moments, your exhale will be naturally longer than your inhale.
- Continue with this breathing pattern for twelve breaths or longer, counting on the inner digits of your hand in a circle as explained in "Counting Your Breaths."
- When you are finished, sit quietly and breathe naturally for a few moments before getting up. ◊

MEDITATION PRACTICE

Moonlight Reflection

The moon and water have been connected with women throughout history. Water is associated with femininity and is symbolically seen as a giver of life. The first life forms on earth evolved in the waters of our oceans just as your baby is developing in the waters of your womb.

Women's cycles are intimately connected to the phases of the moon, which also influence the tides of the ocean. The moon's gravitational power pulls the waters in the ocean and has the ability to affect the waters in your body. A woman's *shakti*, her power, nurturing spirit, and fertility, is associated with the moon as well. Classical Ayurvedic texts advise pregnant woman to bathe in the moonlight.

This meditation can inspire and help connect you to the power, beauty, and radiance of the moon and water. As you are guided to bring their luminosity within, you can also tap into your intuitive, feminine self.

- Sit in a comfortable position, either in Sukhasana on a cushion or in a chair. If you prefer to lie down on your back, use pillows for support under your knees. If you are returning to this meditation in the second and third trimesters and wish to lie on your side, use pillows under your head and your belly.
- Take a few deep and relaxed breaths to settle in, then let your breath be natural. Relax your shoulders.
- Close your eyes. Let your attention turn inward.
- Now visualize yourself by a natural body of water—a lake, a river, or an ocean. See yourself standing by the edge of one of these—such as a pristine mountain lake, gently flowing river, or a calm ocean. The moon is full, glowing brightly above you and reflecting in the water in front of you.
- Slowly make your way into the safe water. Feel the absolute perfect temperature of the water—not too hot and not too cold. Swim into the reflection of the moonlight.
- Bask in the brightness of the full moon as you float in the warm water. Embrace your changing body and feel your baby evolving inside.
- Dunk your head back and let the water renew and refresh your spirit. Feel the moon's glowing and nourishing essence energize and

uplift you. Let the lunar energy draw out your natural inner source of strength and knowing. Find comfort in the moonlight and peace from the water.

- If your mind wanders, focus on your breath. Let each breath connect you back to the water and the moon.
- Keep swimming safely in the warm, natural waters, basking in the brightness of the moonlight and connecting within.
- Now make your way back to the water's edge and slowly get out of the water. Wrap yourself in a large towel, sit down by the water's edge, and thank the moon and water for sharing this experience with you.
- Begin to notice the sounds of the room around you. Gradually open your eyes and sit quietly for a few moments before getting up. ◊

SOUND PRACTICE

Mantra Pushpam

"Mantra Pushpam" is a very long chant honoring water as a nurturing force that ancient seers believed was responsible for creation. This chant speaks about visualizing flowers growing from water, just as your baby is growing from the waters inside of you. "Mantra Pushpam" is often chanted by pregnant women and those who wish to conceive.

- Sit in a comfortable position.
- For each of the following phrases, take a natural breath in, then exhale, reciting one line per exhale:

Yo pam (yo paam)
Pushpam veda (pushpaam vedaa)
Pushpavan prajavan (push-paa-vaan pra-ja-vaan)
Pashuman bhavati (pa-shu-maan bha-va-tee)
Yo pam pushpam veda
Pushpavan prajavan, pashuman bhavati

- Recite the last two lines three more times.
- When finished, sit quietly for a few moments before getting up. ◊

Month Two

PROTECTION

The best protection any woman can have . . . is courage.
ELIZABETH CADY STANTON

It's natural for pregnant women to feel vulnerable, especially in the first trimester. The first three months are a delicate time of adjusting to the pregnancy, hormonal shifts, body sensations, excitement, anxiety, and other emotions. On top of all this, many women experience morning sickness, which is a catchall term for nausea, queasiness, and vomiting, that is not limited to the morning time.

Morning sickness is a telltale sign of pregnancy. It usually begins around six weeks, and can last until the fourteenth week. It is rare for it to last the entire pregnancy. *Morning sickness is a completely normal and healthy response to pregnancy*. No one knows exactly what causes it, even though it has been studied thoroughly.

Some scientists suggest that morning sickness provides a protective mechanism for the developing embryo. A woman's sensitivities to foods and their odors prevent her from consuming substances that could potentially harm the baby. The most common foods women have aversions to are fish, meat, poultry, and some vegetables. Perhaps women evolved to create these disinclinations since ancient times, when bacteria and parasites easily contaminated animal foods. Nausea and vomiting can also occur from overeating, which we sometimes do when intense hunger hits. While no one wants to suffer, morning sickness may have a favorable outcome, as women who experience it tend to have lower risks of miscarriage.

From an Ayurvedic perspective, morning sickness is due to an aggravation of the Pitta dosha. The functions of estrogen are governed by Pitta. Rising estrogen levels in the blood during pregnancy can trigger Pitta in the stomach and increase acidic secretions. This tends to happen in the morning, when the stomach is empty and more acidic.

According to Ayurveda, the earth element is especially dominant in pregnancy. The earth element is responsible for the growth, solidity, and structure of the fetus. The sense of smell is also associated with the earth element. Perhaps this is why pregnant women are especially sensitive to smells. I remember feeling hypersensitive to odors—especially to wafts of garlic cooking when I entered a restaurant—even before I took the pregnancy test for my first pregnancy. Strong odors can trigger nausea and vomiting during pregnancy. Many women try to stay home as much as possible in the first trimester to help control their environment a little more when they are extra sensitive.

I didn't experience any morning sickness in my first pregnancy, but in my second it was quite bothersome. When I was researching the classical Ayurvedic texts, I found many of the suggestions referred to ingredients that were difficult to find in the Western world and quite foreign to me, as a Western woman. A world-renowned Ayurvedic physician once suggested burning a peacock feather and consuming its ash with honey to alleviate morning sickness. While I am always open to Ayurvedic remedies from the ancient past, that one was beyond what I was willing to do. I settled on fresh ginger tea, crackers, coconut water, and a little of the herb shatavari, which really did quell my first trimester nausea and also quieted my mind. Treating morning sickness is covered in appendix 1, "Remedies for Common Pregnancy Ailments."

Shatavari: A Gift for Women

Shatavari is an extraordinary Ayurvedic herb for women, especially during preconception, pregnancy, postpartum, and menopause. It is deeply nourishing to the mother and fetus and can help alleviate morning sickness, heartburn, and indigestion, and improve lactation, among other benefits.

To use it, mix 1 teaspoon in 1 cup of warm, spiced milk (see page 219) or in a small amount of warm water. You can also take in tablets or other classical preparations, such as shatavari ghee or shatavari rasayana. *However, women who experience signs of estrogen dominance such as fibrocystic breasts or uterine fibroids should err on the side of caution and not take this powerful herb. It is also not good for high Kapha.*

See the resources section for where to purchase shatavari.

Using Milk in Pregnancy

The classical Ayurvedic texts advise women to drink milk throughout pregnancy, especially in the first trimester when many women experience nausea and vomiting, to prevent dehydration and supply nourishment. Ayurveda views milk as purely sattvic by nature and a complete, wholesome food in itself. However, contemporary health circles often give milk a bad rap. It's essential to look at its benefits and how it is consumed and produced, and not necessarily blame milk itself.

Milk is anabolic (building, not reducing) and especially nourishes the deeper tissues of the body, such as the reproductive organs (*shukra dhatu*), from which ojas (the essence of the immune system) is created. Milk supports the strength of bones and teeth and can fortify the nervous system. Milk provides abundant calcium and protein, which are vital in pregnancy. If milk agrees with you (does not cause bloating, gas, congestion, or diarrhea), you can enjoy this rich, nutritive food—if it is properly prepared.

Preparation is key! When fresh organic milk is gently warmed, mildly spiced, and taken without other foods, it becomes an elixir of health. This is quite different than using nonorganic milk taken cold right from the refrigerator and pouring it on cereal first thing in the morning, or drinking it by large glassfuls with meals. Milk served in this way can lead to congestion and possibly food allergies, obesity, and heart disease, among other conditions. One of my beloved teachers of Ayurveda, Bri Maya Tiwari, has always said that milk is one food that has been used widely, but not wisely.

Quantity is also essential. Generally, Vata types can enjoy more milk than Kapha types. The type of milk is also essential. Vata types benefit from whole milk—the extra fat helps cushion the nerves. Two percent is ideal for Pitta types, and Kapha types can enjoy 1% or skim milk.

Spices warm up the cold nature of milk, making it lighter and more digestible and dispelling its mucus-forming tendencies. Typical spices

Shatavari Rasayana

Rasayana means "rejuvenation." This preparation of shatavari will help to build up your tissues, nourish the fetus, increase breast milk production, and reduce hyperacidity.

Ingredients

1 pinch saffron threads
½ cup ghee
2 cups shatavari powder
1 cup unrefined sugar, such as sucanat
1 pinch powdered cardamom

Directions

Soak saffron threads in a small amount of water for a couple minutes, then drain.

Heat ghee in a large skillet. When melted and hot, add remaining ingredients and the drained saffron threads. Keep stirring until you can smell their aromas and the mixture is light brown.

Let cool and store in a glass jar.

Take 1 teaspoon daily.

include combinations of cardamom, turmeric, cinnamon, and small amounts of ginger and nutmeg. A touch of honey added after warming it will also balance the qualities of milk.

Warm, spiced milk imbibed before bedtime promotes sound, deep sleep and is in fact an effective treatment for insomnia. Add a teaspoon of ghee and it is an excellent, safe remedy for constipation. Milk blended with almonds, dates, and a pinch of cardamom in the morning or early afternoon is a superb energy and ojas booster.

Where milk comes from matters. The nonorganic commercial milk (and meat) industry is very inhumane and environmentally damaging. It goes against the principle of nonviolence toward all beings, including animals. Milk in its unadulterated form (neither pasteurized nor homogenized), straight from the cow, is not available to many of us today, but fresh milk from organic farms does possess the purity and good intentions present in raw milk. Buy milk and dairy products from organic farms that are local, if possible. It is a worthy investment that benefits the cows, you, your community, and Mother Earth. If it is not available to you, or if you are lactose intolerant, you can use milk substitutes such as almond or rice milk for Vata; almond, soy, or rice milk for Pitta; and soy or rice milk for Kapha types. Fresh goat milk is less mucus-forming than cow's milk and is a good tridoshic option for those who are sensitive to cow's milk.

JOURNALING EXERCISE

Acknowledging and Releasing Fears

Fear can creep up on even the most confident woman in the world. Use this opportunity to explore your fears about this pregnancy and motherhood, no matter how strange or unfounded they may seem.

Part 1: Set aside quiet, undisturbed time and write down all the fears and anxieties in your mind right now. Get them out of your head and onto paper. Make your list as long as it needs to be.

For example:

- I'm afraid I will feel sick for nine months and won't enjoy my pregnancy at all.
- I'm afraid of the pain of giving birth.

- I'm worried that my partner won't be attracted to me when I gain
  weight in pregnancy.
- I'm scared to become a mother.

Part 2: Go outside on a day that's not windy. Light a match to your list.
As it burns, watch the smoke carry your fears away. Then say an affirmation
relative to your statement. For example, if you wrote, "I'm afraid of the pain
of giving birth," you could say, "I'm confident in my strength to give birth to
my baby, and I have the reserves to handle what comes my way."

BREATHING PRACTICE

Shitali Pranayama

Laura had been practicing yoga for ten years. She experienced a lot of
morning sickness in the first trimester, which affected her ability to practice yoga. Every forward bend and forward movement made her feel like
she was going to throw up. She became frustrated because yoga was a big
part of her life and a needed respite from her busy day. After talking with
her about the whole scope of yoga practice, I suggested that she take a
break from asana for a short time. I asked her to go for a brisk walk and
upon returning, practice shitali pranayama with meditation. I also suggested she make some changes to her diet. After a few weeks on her new
program, she felt tremendously better, physically and mentally. Her morning sickness was not completely gone, but she was able to function much
better in all aspects of her life.

Shitali comes from the Sanskrit word meaning "cooling" or "soothing." Based on its name, you can imagine what this breathing practice
does: it reduces heat in the body by cooling and calming the bodily systems and the mind. Some women find this works well for first trimester
morning sickness.

This breathing practice asks you to curl your tongue. The ability to curl
the tongue is a genetic trait, not something that can be learned. If you are
not able to curl your tongue, don't worry; instead, simply place the tip of
your tongue behind your two front teeth.

- Sit in a comfortable position. You can sit cross-legged on the floor,
  on a cushion in Sukhasana, or in a chair.

- Take a deep breath and let your breath elongate your spine. Keep your shoulders relaxed.
- Make an *O* shape with your mouth. Curl your tongue if you are able, or place your tongue behind your two front teeth.
- Inhale slowly and gently lift your chin (avoid throwing your head back). You will feel cold air coming into your mouth. It is as if your curled tongue were a straw, and you're sucking the air in through it.
- When you finish inhaling, close your mouth. Exhale slowly through your nose, and lower your head back to a neutral position.
- Continue inhaling and exhaling in this manner at your own pace. Slowly repeat for a total of twelve breaths, counting on the digits of your hand as explained in chapter 6 (see "Counting Your Breaths" on page 84).
- When you are finished, sit quietly and breathe naturally for a few moments before getting up. 💧

MEDITATION PRACTICE

Protection

This meditation can help increase feelings of being protected. You may enjoy this meditation before you go out into the world; for example, in the morning before going to work.

- Sit in a comfortable position. You can sit cross-legged on the floor, on a cushion in Sukhasana, or in a chair.
- Close your eyes. Relax your shoulders. Relax your body.
- Take several slow, deep breaths to bring your awareness to your life force—your breath, your prana.
- Feel the breath move in through your nostrils. Feel the breath move out of your nostrils.
- Visualize a protective field all around you, like a soft yet thick invisible layer or bubble. This field filters what's helpful from what's harmful so that only what is beneficial is around you. Positivity and all its related emotions (happiness, serenity, protection) are inside with you. Fear cannot penetrate the protective field.
- Let your breath naturally rise and fall as you link to the security,

stability, and strength of feeling protected. Visualize and feel your whole being safeguarded.

- Allow yourself to connect to any other personal associations with feelings of protection.
- As you inhale, silently say to yourself: "I am protected. My baby is protected. My family is protected." Exhale naturally. Repeat these sentences with each in-breath as you draw in the feeling of the phrase: "I am protected. My baby is protected. My family is protected."
- Repeat the affirmation once more, for a total of three times. If your awareness wanders, gently bring it back to your breath and the affirmation.
- When you are finished, sit quietly and breathe naturally for a few moments. Notice the sounds around you and gradually open your eyes before getting up. ●

SOUND PRACTICE

Devi Sureshvari

This sound practice is taken from a longer chant called "Song to the Ganga," which is a prayer to the Goddess. The song in its entirety has a beautiful melody. The last line translates to, "Give your protection from my ignorance, one whose nature is compassion."

- Sit in a comfortable position. You can sit cross-legged on the floor, on a cushion in Sukhasana, or in a chair.
- For each of the following phrases, take a natural breath in, then exhale, reciting one line per exhale:

Pahi (paa-hee)
Krpa-mayi (kripaa-maayee)
Mama-jnanam (maa-mah-gnyaa-nahm)
Pahi krpa-mayi
Mama-jnanam
Pahi krpa-mayi mama-jnanam

- When finished, sit quietly for a few moments before getting up. ●

Month Three

PEACE

Peace begins with a smile.
MOTHER TERESA

I remember self-image issues surfacing around the third month in both my pregnancies when I started to feel plump and my clothes were becoming snug. I was not ready for the world to know I was pregnant. Psychologically, I did not want to wear maternity clothes yet. I purchased a few pairs of yoga pants larger than I usually wear. They looked good, were so comfortable, and nobody knew I was pregnant. Most of all, I felt at ease and at peace with how my body was changing because I could integrate my pregnancy at my own pace and I didn't feel self-conscious anymore. These pants stretched with me during the entire course of my pregnancies, and I wore them through the postpartum time. Then I retired the pants and didn't want to look at them ever again!

Gaining weight is a point of contention for countless women. Scores of women wish they were thinner, while others cannot gain weight even if they try. Our modern culture, the media, and especially the advertising and fashion industries contribute immensely to these issues. Different body types have distinctive body structures, contrasting metabolisms, and emotional tendencies. All women during pregnancy need extra calories, regardless of doshic type. Weight gain and where you carry your extra weight will be different for every woman. Your pre-pregnancy weight, body mass index (BMI), and activity level need to be taken into consideration as well.

Vata types can gain weight on the higher side during pregnancy, since they are often underweight from the beginning and can afford to put on more weight than other types. But their erratic appetite can also prevent them from gaining adequate weight. Pitta women usually have average weight gain. Kapha types can go to either extreme. While it is easier for the Kapha woman to put on a lot of extra weight due to her Kapha nature (food preferences and tendency to be lethargic when it comes to activity), she may also enter pregnancy on the heavier side and may not need to gain much at all.

Listen to your appetite; eat when you are hungry and stop when you are satisfied. As long as you are eating a healthy, well-balanced variety of foods and enjoying dosha-appropriate exercise relative to pregnancy, *you should not be concerned with weight gain*. Your body and your baby's development depend on it! In the nineteenth century and early twentieth century, women were told to restrict their food intake to limit weight gain. This false premise was based on the idea that it is easier to deliver a smaller baby than a larger one. Following the recommendation led to many low birth weight babies, with delayed neurological development and with greater risks of developing infections. Now it has been proven that healthy weight gain leads to healthy babies. While there is no one-size-fits-all approach, women typically gain twenty to thirty-five pounds in a normal pregnancy, based on the factors mentioned above. Work with your prenatal care provider to discover what's right for you.

Where all the weight comes from (approximately):

Baby, 7 ½ pounds
Placenta, 1 ½ pounds
Amniotic fluid, 2 pounds
Uterine enlargement, 2 pounds
Mother's breast tissue, 2 pounds
Mother's blood, 4 pounds
Fluids in mother's tissues, 4 pounds
Mother's fat stores, 7 pounds
Average total: 30 pounds

Perhaps the best advice for addressing the weight and body-image issues that can surface during pregnancy comes from the book *Ina May's Guide to Childbirth* by the nation's leading midwife, Ina May Gaskin: "Even if it has not been your habit throughout your life so far, I recommend that you learn to think positively about your body."

JOURNALING EXERCISE

Accepting Your Changing Body as Healthy

Accepting your changing body as healthy, perfect, and complete sets the stage for a more peaceful and enjoyable pregnancy. The concept of *isvara pranidahana* from the yoga sutras illuminates the idea of letting go of pre-conceived notions. In your pregnancy, this relates to what you think you "should" look like. Isvara pranidahana is surrendering to what is beyond us, which includes Mother Nature's process. Cultivating this attitude is not only essential for your baby's health, but also a key element for creating a sattvic mind.

Ask yourself, "What do I feel when I look at myself in the mirror? What do I love about my body? What do I wish was different?" If your feelings are positive, enjoy them and let this exercise uplift you. If your feelings are negative or critical, use this opportunity to replace them with a positive message. Make time to write freely and honestly about these ideas. For example:

Critical thought: *Fat* is the only word to describe how I feel right now. I can't imagine how I'll feel in six months.

Positive message: I have waited to see my belly grow with a baby for two years now. I can't believe it's actually happening! I love to see it finally pop out.

Critical thought: I wish my thighs and bottom didn't look so large.

Positive message: I think I'm starting to look like those goddess images of beautiful round, full women.

When you are finished, ask yourself if you feel more at peace with your changing body. ◗

BREATHING PRACTICE

Ujjayi Pranayama

This pranayama practice is a balancing and calming technique that encourages the free and healthy flow of prana. The sound made during *ujjayi* breathing can help you focus your mind on your breath. Ujjayi is usually done during asana practice but can also be used while sitting in preparation for meditation. The key to working with this technique is simply to relax.

- Sit in a comfortable position. You can sit cross-legged on the floor, on a cushion in Sukhasana, or in a chair.
- Take a deep breath and let that breath lengthen your spine. Keep your eyes closed. Never force your breath; be gentle with it.
- Inhale through your nose, and then *slowly* exhale through your open mouth.
- Do this again: inhale through your nose, and then slowly exhale through your open mouth. As the air moves through the back of your throat, it makes a *ha* sound.
- Repeat this breath a couple of times, and then close your mouth.
- Now, with your mouth closed, inhale and exhale through your nose and direct the breath slowly across the back of your throat. This should create an ocean sound—like ocean waves crashing on the shore.
- Practice twelve full, long, and smooth repetitions—a full repetition is an inhale and exhale. You can count on the digits of your hand as explained in chapter 6 (see "Counting Your Breaths," page 84).
- Return to your natural breathing before getting up.

MEDITATION PRACTICE

Focusing the Mind, Encouraging Peace (So Hum)

So Hum meditation is a wonderful contemplative practice, as it is easy to connect each breath to the *so hum* sounds. In fact, the sounds of *so hum* actually reflect the natural sounds of the breath. You can hear the *so* sound subtly in each inhale, and the *hum* in each exhale. After over fifteen years of meditation, I still frequently return to this practice for its simple ability to quiet the mind and to evoke joyful feelings of peace.

- Sit comfortably on a cushion in Sukhasana, or in a chair. Alternatively, use blankets and pillows to make yourself comfortable.
- Take a deep breath. Let your breath lengthen your spine. Slightly tuck your chin to allow the back of your neck to lengthen.
- Place your hands on your lap with your palms facing up. Relax your shoulders.
- Close your eyes and bring your awareness to your breath. Keep your mouth closed and breathe through your nose. Take a few moments to observe the flow of your inhalation and exhalation.
- Once you are comfortable watching your breath, silently say the word *so* to yourself with each inhale. Say the word *hum* with each exhale.
- Practice twelve repetitions, counted on the inner digits of your hand as explained in chapter 6 (see "Counting Your Breaths," page 84). Allow yourself to be drawn inward as you move into deeper rhythm with *so hum*.
- If your mind wanders, use the words to gently bring your focus back to your breath and the syllables *so* and *hum*.
- When you are finished, sit quietly for a few moments in the silence of your meditation before getting up. Allow the peace to stay with you as you move on to other activities.

Once you are familiar with this practice, you can go for as long as you like or set a timer for yourself for five or ten minutes. If you would like to refine the practice and add another element of focus, see if you can match the length of your inhale with the length your silent recitation of *so*, and match the length of your exhale with the length of your silent recitation of *hum*. Practice making the inhaled *so* and the exhaled *hum* the same length a few times, until it becomes natural for you. ◗

SOUND PRACTICE
Shanti, Shanti, Shanti

Shanti means "peace," "calm," or "serenity" in Sanskrit. The sound itself is just as beautiful as its meaning.

Begin this exercise with a strong voice that progressively gets softer as you add more peace onto the chant.

- Sit in a comfortable position with your back straight. You can sit cross-legged on the floor, on a cushion in Sukhasana, or in a chair.
- For each of the following phrases, take a natural breath in, then exhale, reciting one line per exhale:

Shantih (shanteehee)
Shanti, shantih (shantee shanteehee)
Shanti, shanti, shantih (shantee shantee shanteehee)

- Now progressively get softer: Om shanti, shanti, shantih
- A little softer: Om shanti, shanti, shantih
- Finally super soft: Om shanti, shanti, shantih
- When finished, sit quietly for a few moments before getting up. Allow the peace to stay with you as you move on to other activities. ◊

9

The Second Trimester

There is something very satisfactory about being in the middle of something.
Marilyn Hacker

Many women let out a huge sigh of relief when they enter their second trimester. The dissipation of nausea and vomiting is a welcomed sign of this new phase of pregnancy. Fears tend to be washed away as the pregnancy is less vulnerable and more established now. Energy and vitality usually increase, bringing a renewed sense of well-being. Your baby is still growing rapidly, but not yet uncomfortably crowding your body. For all these reasons, this was my favorite stage in both of my pregnancies.

What's Happening in Your Body?

The following sections present general information on your baby's growth and development and typical physical and emotional changes during this trimester. This is not an exhaustive list and there are always variations within the normal range. Every woman's experience of pregnancy is unique, whether it is your first or your fifth. Also, please keep in mind that there is an immeasurable element of mystery during pregnancy that continually creates new experiences.

The fetus is making more strides as the soft cartilage in the skeleton begins to become bone. The kidneys start to function, allowing your baby to create urine and discharge it into the amniotic fluid. Fingernails, toenails, eyelashes, and eyebrows form. Hair begins to grow on his head, and lanugo, a soft fine hair, covers his shoulders, back, and temples. He can even suck his thumb, yawn, stretch, and make faces.

After sixteen weeks, the reproductive organs and genitalia are fully developed. An ultrasound can reveal the baby's sex, if this is something you wish to know. Ayurvedic pulse diagnosis can also uncover the sex. There is a special pulse at the base and inner side of the pinky finger. If a strong pulse is felt on the right side, the fetus is male. If a strong pulse is felt on the left side, the fetus is female. Feel for a pulse on both sides and the more prominent pulse will become clear. I have been surprised by the accuracy of this pulse. Clients and friends often challenge me to determine their baby's gender, and all but once I have been correct. It's fun to play around and experiment with this even if you are not trained in pulse diagnosis.

By eighteen weeks the fetus can hear sounds, such as your voice, heart beating, and stomach growling, as well as sounds outside your body. He may soon be able to respond to familiar sounds with movements. You may feel a fluttery sensation at first that can be difficult to recognize. As your pregnancy progresses, the movements will become more obvious. The fetus's heartbeat is also now audible, and listening to it for the first time is very exciting.

TYPICAL PHYSICAL CHANGES

Growing belly. The uterus becomes heavier and expands to make room for the baby, which causes your abdomen to expand. You may gain three to four pounds a month until delivery; this weight gain is beneficial, healthy, and necessary.

Leg cramps. Your leg muscles may become tired from carrying extra weight, and pressure from the uterus can impede blood flow to the legs, causing leg cramps. Calcium and magnesium deficiencies can also cause leg muscles to cramp.

Dizziness. Your blood vessels dilate due to pregnancy hormones. Until your blood volume expands to fill them, your blood pressure may fall and you might experience dizziness. Make sure you are drinking plenty of fluids and rising slowly after lying or sitting down.

Vaginal secretions. You may experience a thin, white vaginal discharge that is thought to help suppress the growth of potentially harmful bacteria and yeast. This is normal.

Skin changes. Certain areas of your skin may become darker, such as around your nipples, parts of your face, and the line that runs from the navel to the pubic bone. This is caused by increased blood circulation to your skin and changing hormonal levels. Your skin is also more sensitive to sun exposure.

Congestion. As your circulation increases, more blood flows through your body's mucous membranes. This causes the lining of your nose and airway to swell, which can restrict airflow, leading to congestion, nosebleeds, and snoring.

Gum problems. Increased blood circulation can soften your gums, making them tender and swollen, and can cause bleeding.

TYPICAL EMOTIONAL CHANGES

As your belly grows, the pregnancy may seem more real than before. Changes in your body's shape and function are continuous reminders of what is happening inside. This trimester can be an opportunity to settle into your pregnancy and feel comfortable. Shopping for maternity clothes can be a fun activity and helps acknowledge these wonderful changes in your body.

Overall, emotions tend to even out in the second trimester, as fatigue lessens and energy picks up. Use this time wisely, as your energy can shift again, once you enter the last trimester. You may now feel more ready for prenatal yoga and other forms of exercise. You may feel inspired to prepare for your baby's arrival and begin to read about breastfeeding, vaccines, circumcision, and other contemporary issues that require careful thought.

Some women feel an increase in their libido during this stage. Others feel unattractive because of their growing belly and are not interested in sex. Try to maintain open communication with your partner about these issues. Your partner or the close friend you've chosen to help you through pregnancy and birth may feel more connected to your pregnancy if they go with you to your prenatal visits. This can help them share in your excitement, anxieties, and dreams for the baby.

In the first half of pregnancy, women are often confronted with decisions about prenatal testing. While this topic is beyond the scope of this book, it's important to take your time researching the pros and cons and discussing them with your prenatal care provider. You may wish to read the prenatal care section of *The Natural Pregnancy Book* by Aviva Romm for a great overview of prenatal testing. Be sure to talk freely with your care provider about anything you are experiencing, even if it seems silly or unimportant. This will help your mind rest easier. If your prenatal care provider seems unresponsive to your concerns, consider switching so that you feel completely cared for in your pregnancy.

10

Month Four

NURTURING

A woman in harmony with her spirit is like a river flowing. She goes where she will without pretense and arrives at her destination prepared to be herself and only herself.
MAYA ANGELOU

Women, especially mothers, have the innate wiring to nurture and nourish other beings. Since the beginning of time, the caregiver role has come naturally to women. Whether you choose a high-powered career or prefer to stay at home with your children, you still possess instinctive nurturing skills. If you have not considered yourself to be a nurturer in the past, pregnancy can be an opportunity to arouse this instinct, leading you into a harmonious relationship with your children. The verb *nurture* is defined in Webster's dictionary as "to supply with nourishment; educate; to further the development of." It comes from the Latin word *nutritus*, meaning "to suckle or nourish."

I never truly understood the word *nurture* until I became a mother. When I nurture my family, I give unconditionally from a deep place within myself. Giving freely from the heart allows me to truly enjoy giving, and witnessing my gifts being received is equally satisfying. There is something particularly fulfilling about encouraging my children to engage in wholesome activities and watching them eat nourishing foods that I lovingly prepare for them. I love to see them gobble up brown rice, steamed broccoli and carrots, and avocados, and shove sheets of nori seaweed in their mouths. They have no idea how much eating these foods deeply sustains them on so many levels, builds up their tissues, and creates healthy eating preferences—hopefully for a lifetime. I cherish the times when they explore simple objects from nature (such as rocks, sand, and water), which nurtures their creativity, and when they read books with hidden positive messages, which subtly nurtures the development of optimism in their lives.

As much as I enjoy endless giving, I also did not realize the importance of nurturing myself until I stepped into my mothering role. The fulfillment and enrichment inherent to motherhood are coupled with exhaustion and depletion, especially if you are committed to conscious parenting. To sustain your own wellness, equilibrium, and happiness, it is essential to nurture yourself in various ways.

JOURNALING EXERCISE

Nurturing Yourself

As a woman, you need to take in much more than food to grow vibrantly. When you feed yourself from a variety of sources—including relaxation, laughter, and good company—you move toward wholeness and replenishment. Giving to others is effortless when you give from a place of deep nourishment.

Take out your journal and ask yourself:

- Do I feel nurtured?
- What helps me to feel nurtured? What activities, relationships, and/ or experiences contribute to my being supported, joyful, and balanced?
- Do I notice a connection between feeling nurtured and nourished and an ease of giving, either to others like my family, or to the greater world?
- How do I feel or act when I don't feel nurtured and nourished?

Write down whatever comes to your mind. Maybe you enjoy taking a long walk with a dear friend and sharing everything that's on your mind, soaking in a hot bath surrounded by candles, or staying in your pajamas until noon.

Now think about how you can make time for these special activities, and make it a priority to include one thing a week or a day, depending upon the amount of time you have.

You may think of a number of reasons to not take time for yourself—you are too busy, can't afford it, it's too complicated. But pregnancy is your time to indulge. Schedule the massage you've wanted to get, or make a lunch date with a girlfriend. It definitely won't be as easy once the baby comes. If this is your first pregnancy, these questions may not seem necessary, but they will probably strike a chord if you already have children.

When I revisited this journaling exercise, I realized that generally I do feel nurtured in my life, but not always as much as I would like. Taking a hike with a close girlfriend in the mountains is at the top of my list of things that make me feel nurtured. I wish I could take these hikes more often. Another simple act that feeds my soul is simply being alone in my home (a nurturing space in itself), diving into a novel while sipping my favorite tea. I am grateful for some time away from my family and work, when I can savor quietness and tranquility.

Nurturing the Cravings and Desires of the Mother

Several classical Ayurvedic texts discuss the desires of a pregnant woman, who is referred to as a *dauhrdini* (literally "two hearted") because she now possesses two hearts. It is said that the fetus attains the free flow of consciousness in the mind when the sense organs are manifested, which is usually in the fourth month. After this time, the fetus can express desires that are connected to the mother's heart and are transmitted through it. Although this has not been scientifically proven, it is suggested that mothers not ignore these desires, because they are actually messages from the fetus about something it needs; in other words, a mother's cravings are nature's way of signaling a need for certain nutrients or experiences. For example, a woman may crave eating the proverbial pickles and ice cream, or wearing silky garments, or spending time by a river.

These texts state that if a pregnant woman fulfills her desires during pregnancy, she will deliver a powerful child that will live a long life. If she does not, she will give birth to a child that will suffer from diseases of the concerned sense organ, with all sorts of bizarre deformities. This is not meant to instill fear in you *at all*, but to elucidate the importance of listening to your heart and deeper desires, even if the rational mind cannot comprehend the yearning. Try out this advice for yourself by indulging in your cravings, as long as they will not harm your or your baby's health.

When I was pregnant with my daughter, I had an overwhelming desire for goat cheese. I would wake up at three in the morning and crave goat Gouda cheese on crackers! Never before had I treasured this snack, yet it became a staple of mine during this pregnancy. Maybe my baby was craving more protein, calcium, or fat? It's hard to know. But before she was two years old she began saying, "More goat cheese please, Mommy!" and it is still one of her favorite things to eat. When I was pregnant with my son, I felt a strong yearning to swim frequently and eat juicy, sweet fruits every day. The desire was so strong that to feed these cravings, I convinced my husband to use our frequent flier miles to go to Hawaii during the sixth month. I was in heaven swimming in the warm ocean waters and devouring the freshest pineapples and papayas I had ever eaten. My son was born under the Western astrological water sign of Cancer, the crab. As I write this, he just turned one year old, and goes absolutely bonkers for peaches, cherries, and other fruit. He also adores the water. Again, it is difficult to ascertain the exact meaning behind the cravings, but they seemed to feed some deep need in both my children and me.

Nurturing Practice: Warm Lavender Baths

This nurturing practice includes turning off your phone, closing your bathroom door, and putting on your absolute favorite soothing or soulful music. Fill the bathtub with warm water. If you are feeling achy, stiff, or sore in any way, add 2 cups of Epsom salts (available from any drug store) or your favorite bath salts. Light a few candles or dim the lights. When the water is drawn, add 10 drops of pure lavender essential oil. Lavender oil is good for all body types and is deeply soothing, calming, and nurturing, among many other benefits. Use your hand to disperse the oils and mix in the salts. Get in and slowly inhale the aromas as you unwind and relax. Splash the warm water over your belly. Take several deep, relaxing breaths. Place your hands on your belly and send the calmness down to your baby. Enjoy this nurturing practice in the evening before bed, or whenever you can give yourself time to relax. It is also lovely after a self-massage.

ASANA PRACTICE

Beginning a Home Prenatal Yoga Practice

The fourth month is an excellent time to dive into asana practice since most women begin to feel better as their pregnancy is established and energy increases. Please reread chapter 2, "The Complete Practice of Yoga," to refresh your mind about the fundamental principles of prenatal yoga.

Following is a simple basic sequence for home practice. Each subsequent chapter for months five through nine of pregnancy will present a new sequence, with some of these poses and some new ones. Always rest in between asanas as needed, especially if you're feeling fatigued, lightheaded, or dizzy, or if you notice any spotting or cramping.

1. TADASANA (MOUNTAIN POSE)

- Stand with legs hip-width apart or wider and your feet facing forward.
- Feel your feet planted firmly on the ground. Your chin is gently tucked and your shoulders are relaxed. Make sure your knees are soft and not locked. Keep your eyes open.
- Place your palms on your belly to send loving thoughts to your baby. Take a few comfortable and relaxed breaths. Feel your belly expand with each inhalation and gently relax with each exhalation.
- Relax your arms by your side.
- Inhale and sweep your arms out to the side and up by your ears. Very slightly arch your back as you look at your hands above your head.
- Exhale and lower your arms back down by your sides. Lower your chin.
- Repeat this arm movement two to three times at your own pace. Link your breath with your movement.
- Now, as you inhale and lift your arms, gradually lift your heels off the floor and come onto the balls of your feet. You don't need to lift your heels up too high, just slightly. Focusing your gaze on something in front of you or on a point on the floor will help you keep your balance.
- Exhale and lower your arms and your heels back down.
- Repeat this movement two to three times, linking your breath with your movement.

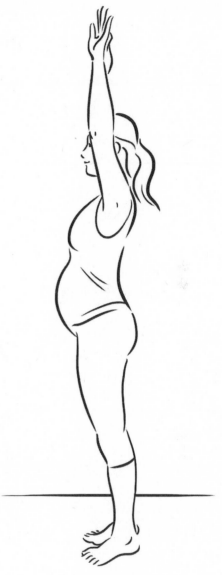

figure 4 **Tadasana** (Mountain Pose)

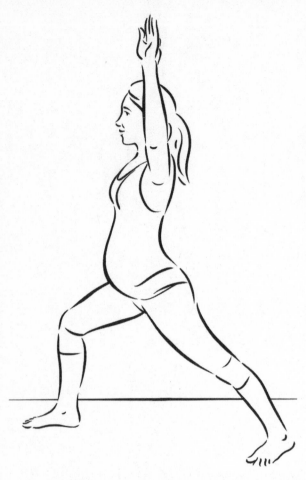

figure 5 **Virabhadrasana**
(Warrior Pose)

2. VIRABHADRASANA (WARRIOR POSE)

- Stand with your legs hip-width apart or wider and your feet facing forward.
- Step your left foot three to four feet forward. Make sure the distance is comfortable for you.
- Turn your right foot slightly out, so your toes point slightly to the right.
- Make sure you have enough width between your legs to feel stable and so that your hips are squared comfortably to the front. Your arms are by your sides.
- As you inhale, bend your left knee and sweep your arms up by your ears. Your weight shifts forward onto your left leg. Lift your chest, gently arching your back.
- As you exhale, lower your arms and straighten your front leg, shifting your weight back.
- Repeat three times. Remember to link your breath to the movement and go at your own pace.
- After three repetitions, step your left foot back, so your feet are together.
- Repeat the sequence on the other side and step your feet together when you're finished.

3. PRASARITA PADOTTANASANA (EXPANDED LEG STRETCH)

For this pose, you may want to have yoga blocks, or a chair with a blanket on it, handy.

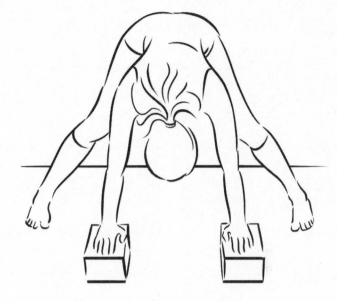

- Standing on your mat lengthwise, start with your feet hip-width apart and your feet facing forward.
- Step your feet three to four feet apart sideways. Make sure your knees are not locked. Rest your arms by your sides.
- As you inhale, lift your arms to bring them by your ears.
- As you exhale, bring your arms down to the top of your thighs, with your palms facing down on your thighs, and bend forward from the hips, sliding your hands down your legs as you finish your exhalation.
- Inhale and slide your hands back up your legs as you bring your torso back upright, returning to the beginning position.
- Do this movement a couple times at your own pace. Move your hands up and down your legs with each inhale and exhale.
- After a few cycles, bend again at the hips and move your hands down your legs. This time, stay in the bottom of the pose (in the forward bend) for several breaths.
- To keep the length in your spine, place your hands on yoga blocks in front of you. Or for a restful, calming effect, rest your elbows and forehead on a blanket-covered chair.
- Keep your awareness on your breath. Breathe into your lower back, the back of your legs, or anywhere that is calling your attention. This pose can allow the baby to move into a more comfortable position as you create more space in your body.
- When you are ready, inhale and lift your torso to come out of the fold. Step your feet together.

figure 6 **Prasarita Padottanasana** (Expanded Leg Stretch)

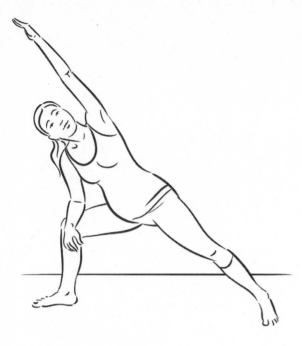

figure 7 **Parshva Konasana**
(Side Angle Pose)

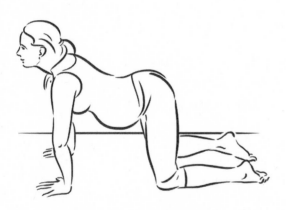

figure 8 **Cakravakasana**
(Ruddy Goose Pose)

4. PARSHVA KONASANA (SIDE ANGLE POSE)

- Start standing, with your legs together, both feet facing forward. Step your legs apart sideways, so they are one leg length apart.
- Turn your right foot ninety degrees to the right and your left foot inward, toward the right, at forty-five degrees.
- Inhale and bring your arms to shoulder height.
- Exhale and, bending your right knee, lunge into your right leg.
- Bring your right forearm to your right thigh. Lift your left arm up, so that it points toward the sky. Your left palm is facing down. Your head is facing forward.
- Breathe into your side body. Inhale and reach through your left fingers to extend the left arm even further.
- Exhale and bend your left elbow, drawing your elbow toward your hip. At the same time, turn your head to look toward the floor.
- Repeat three times: inhale and exhale, moving your arm through space as you turn your head, creating length in your side body.
- Inhale and come out of the pose by bringing your arms back to shoulder height and straightening your right leg. Release your arms to your sides.
- Repeat on the other side.

5. CAKRAVAKASANA (RUDDY GOOSE POSE)

This pose has many variations. Here you will be gently rocking back and forth on your hands and knees to open the spine, chest, and pelvis, which helps to release tension in the head, neck, and spine.

- Start on your hands and knees, with your hands under your shoulders and your knees under your hips or slightly wider than hip-width apart.
- On an inhalation, gently lift your chest and your head away from your belly, lifting your heart center.
- On an exhalation, round your lower back as you bring your hips toward your heels, as far as comfortable, making room for your belly.
- Inhale back up to the starting position.
- Repeat the entire movement cycle three to five more times. Gently link breath and movement as you gently rock back and forth.
- Finish by returning to the neutral starting position.

6. ADHO MUKHA SHVANASANA (DOWNWARD FACING DOG POSE)

- Start on your hands and knees, with your hands directly under your shoulders and your knees directly under your hips.
- Inhale and lift the head and chest.
- Exhale, tuck your toes under, and lift your buttocks up toward the sky. As you do, drop your head toward the earth and straighten your arms and spine. Your heels may or may not come down to the floor. Your legs don't need to straighten. It's more important that your spine is straight than that your legs are.
- Take an in-breath here. Then as you exhale, drop your knees back to the floor.
- Repeat the cycle two more times.
- Once again, from the hands and knees position, inhale and lift your head and chest. As you exhale, tuck your toes under and push your hands into the floor as your straighten your arms, sending your tailbone up to the sky. This time, stay for a few breaths. Keep your awareness on long and smooth breaths.
- When you are ready, drop your knees to the floor to come out of the pose.

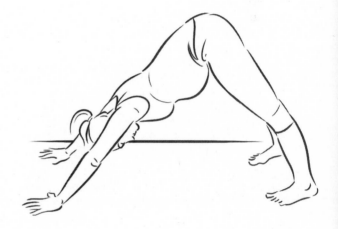

figure 9 **Adho Mukha Shvanasana** (Downward Facing Dog Pose)

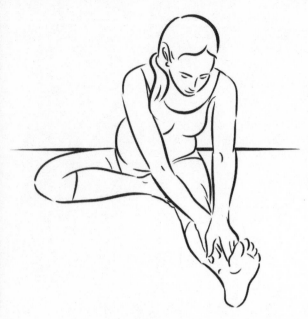

figure 10 **Janu Shirshasana**
(Head to Knee Pose)

7. JANU SHIRSHASANA (HEAD TO KNEE POSE)

Even though this pose is called "Head to Knee," don't try to touch your head to your knee when you're pregnant!

- Sit on your buttocks on the floor and extend your left leg out in front of you. Bring the sole of your right foot to the inner thigh of your left leg.
- Inhale and lift your arms to your ears.
- Exhale and move your chest (heart center) forward from your hips, toward your left foot. Place your hands somewhere on your left leg, thigh, or knee. Only fold down as a far as comfortable and as far as your belly allows.
- Inhale, lift your arms back up to your ears, and to come out of the pose, lift your torso back up to straight.
- Move in and out of the pose two times, linking your breath with the movements. Feel your spine lengthen with each inhale, and stretch your lower back, one side at a time, as you bend forward from your hips, on each exhale.
- The third time you bend forward, stay in the forward bend for a breath or two.
- Inhale, lift your arms to your ears, and lift your torso to come out of the pose again. Lower your arms.
- Switch your legs and repeat the whole sequence on the other side.

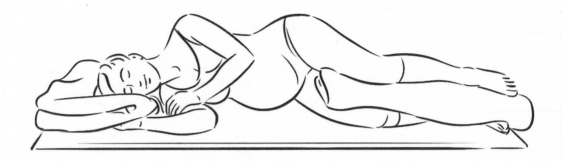

8. SHAVASANA (CORPSE POSE)

You will need a few blankets, or a yoga bolster and one blanket for this pose.

figure 11 **Shavasana** (Corpse Pose)

- Lie on your side, either your left or right, with a blanket or bolster between your thighs and feet, and another blanket under your head. Your knees are relaxed and soft, and your ankles and feet are supported by the blanket.
- Let your breath be natural. Close your eyes and draw your attention inward.
- Mentally scan your body and consciously relax any tense places. Let your whole body feel heavy, as if you were sinking into the floor underneath you.
- Stay in this pose for about five minutes, or until you feel rested and centered.
- To come out of the pose, begin to notice the sounds around you. Begin to feel your breath in your body again. Gently move your fingers and toes. Use your hands and arms to bring yourself slowly back into a seated position. ◆

BREATHING PRACTICE

Shitali Pranayama with Ujjayi Exhale

In this practice, you will combine two types of breathing that you learned in the first trimester. Begin with inhaling in a shitali mouth position, and exhale in ujjayi. They blend well together and lead you into a deeper relationship with your breath.

- Sit in a comfortable position.
- Take a few deep breaths and let your breath elongate your spine. Sit up tall, yet stay relaxed.
- Make an *O* shape with your mouth and curl your tongue, if you are able. If not, simply place the tip of your tongue behind your two front teeth.
- Inhale and feel air moving over your tongue as you slowly and gently lift your chin.
- When you finish, close your mouth; exhale through your nose as you direct the breath slowly across the back of your throat. This should create an ocean sound. Lower your head back to a neutral position while exhaling.
- Continue this breath pattern four or five more times—or more if you wish—at your own pace. Try to create a long and smooth breath. Remember to be gentle with your breath.
- When you are finished, sit for a moment or two to allow your breath to normalize before going on to your next activity. 🌢

MEDITATION PRACTICE

Trataka, Nurturing Yourself with Candlelight

Trataka means "to look" or "gaze," and is a traditional meditation practice where you gaze at a candle flame. This simple practice improves concentration, decreases mental lethargy, and increases *buddhi* (intellect). Trataka brings calmness and tranquility. For pregnant women, the most important aspect of the practice is how it focuses the mind and encourages relaxation. After practicing trataka in your pregnancy, you may use it in early labor to calm and center you.

It's important never to force yourself to gaze in a way that strains your eyes, brain, or body. Gazing will develop naturally over time.

- Place a lit candle at eye level and about one arm's length in front of you. (Make sure there are no strong breezes around.)
- Sit in a comfortable position and try to relax your body as much as possible. Relax your shoulders, and release your jaw and other areas where you tend to hold tension.
- Let your breath be natural.
- Rest your hands on your belly. Close your eyes and take several slow, deep breaths into your belly.
- Now open your eyes and gaze at the brightest point of the flame. Stay focused on the flame. Blink and close your eyes if you need to. Otherwise, keep your eyes open, gazing at the flame. Continue breathing deeply.
- After a couple minutes, close your eyes and observe your breath.
- Then, open your eyes again and gaze at the brightest point of the flame. Keep your awareness on long, smooth breaths into your belly as you focus your eyes and your mind on the candle flame.
- After a couple minutes, close your eyes and observe your breath again.
- When you are finished, sit quietly with your eyes closed for a few minutes before getting up.

This meditation can also be done while relaxing in a warm bath. Place several candles around you and choose one flame to focus on.

SOUND PRACTICE
Ha Vu Ha

"Ha Vu Ha" is taken from a longer chant from the Taittiriya Upanishad. The simplest translation of this is "Oh, wonderful!" As all of pregnancy is a time to increase joy in your life, let this chant lift, lighten, and nourish you. If you chant it in the morning, use more strength in your voice to energize your day. If you chant it before bed, let your voice be soft and slow to prepare yourself for a peaceful slumber.

- Sit in a comfortable position.
- For each of the following phrases, take a natural breath in, then exhale, reciting one line per exhale:

Ha (haa)
Ha vu (haa vuu)
Ha vu ha (haa vuu haa)
Ha vu ha vu (haa vuu haa vuu)
Ha vu ha vu ha (haa vuu haa vuu haa)
Ha vu ha vu ha vu (haa vuu haa vuu haavuuuu)
Ha vu ha

- When finished, sit quietly for a few moments before getting up. ◊

11

Month Five

MOTHERING

The health of every family begins with the mother.
She is the tree from which the healthy fruit must come.
JULIETTE DE BAIRACLI LEVY

One day during my second pregnancy, I was rereading—for the umpteenth time—Juliette de Bairacli Levy's classic text on natural child rearing, *Nature's Children*, and the opening quote evoked a heartfelt resonance. She eloquently touched on the significance of a mother's health as the wellspring for a healthy family. Mothers *are* the reservoirs that provide sustenance and well-being to their families.

To mother a child is one of the most momentous and influential jobs in a woman's life. It is referred to by one of my teachers as a *maha-dharma* or "great duty," above and beyond all other dharmas in life. I am defining *dharma* here as a duty, responsibility, and purpose, which includes career, but also encompasses much more. We have many dharmas throughout our lifetime: dharmas to our society, to our parents, to our spouses or partners, and dharmas to our children. The dharma of motherhood includes serving as a positive role model for your children, guiding and supporting them, building confidence and compassion in them, instilling strong values and ethics, and encouraging their growth and development as individual beings. This is a tall order!

It is natural to contemplate your own experiences with your mother while you are in the process of becoming a mother yourself or evolving as a mother, if you already have children. There is a deep and mysterious bond between mothers and their children, especially their daughters. You are intuitively and intimately connected. I am often reminded of this because I seem to always know when my mother is calling on the phone before I answer the call. I have no idea how this happens, but I get a sense that it is her and it almost always is.

Much is passed down through the maternal line, both positive and negative. You carry the memory of your forbears in your cells—physically, emotionally, and spiritually. This inseparable connection to your past carries joy and heartache, as well as propensities for strength and disease. Women especially benefit from knowing about the health of the women in their family, for as many previous generations as possible. All that you inherit gives you knowledge and understanding about where you come from, which can guide and protect you in the years to come.

To help you become more present in your role as a mother and deepen your own process of healing, you can explore your childhood experiences, especially your relationship to your mother. For some women, this exploration can bring up mixed emotions, but it is an opportunity to get to know another side of your mother and possibly heal wounds and unresolved feelings from the past. It can also be an opening to becoming closer with her before you become a mother and she a grandmother. If your mother is still alive and in contact with you, you can start your exploration by asking her what her pregnancy with you and your birth were like. Ask her what the early years were like for her.

After my children were born, I had this conversation with my mother. Before we spoke, I had my own experiences and feelings about motherhood. As the unspoken became spoken, I discovered uncanny similarities. Both of my labors were similar to both of my mother's in duration and intensity. We both felt strongly about being the primary caregiver for our children, especially in the early years, but also had a compelling need to fulfill other aspects of our lives, such as our work in the world. We both noticed that having something of our own, in addition to motherhood, helped us to feel more balanced. With young children, working a few mornings a week helped each of us to become better, more patient and loving mothers.

The more positive and healthy the relationship between you and your mother is, the freer you feel physically, emotionally, and mentally. Often unresolved issues can create health problems and lead to feelings of frustration and anger. Choosing to clear the air and move through these issues can lead to greater joy and freedom in your life.

There can be times when it is truly unhealthy to be in contact with your mother. For example, if the relationship is unsupportive and there are reasons why you cannot communicate. Then, cultivating compassion and distance may be the most healing for everyone. If your mother has passed away, or if you were adopted and never knew your birth mother, it may be healing to explore these questions with other family members, such as an aunt, father, or close family friend. In these situations, perhaps, there is a mother figure available for you. It can be a personal relationship or even a more distant one with a woman such as a saint or spiritual teacher who nurtures your spirit and supports your life in deep ways.

JOURNALING EXERCISE
What Being a Mother Means to You

Pregnancy is an appropriate time to ponder what it means for you to be or to become a mother. Write down whatever comes to your mind. Use these questions to spark some ideas:

- What qualities do you associate with the word *mother?*
- How would you describe your mother (or the main maternal figure in your life)? What are her positive qualities?
- Did your mother (or other caregiver) create feelings in your childhood home that you want to recreate for your family? What are these?
- What responsibilities will be yours once you become a mother?

ASANA PRACTICE
Pelvic Openings

What better way to prepare for motherhood than to work on opening your pelvis to birth your baby? Women naturally have a wider, more circular

Kegel Exercises

Kegel exercises strengthen the pelvic floor muscles, which naturally weaken from pregnancy and birth. You can identify your pelvic muscles by stopping and starting the flow of urine when going to the bathroom. Once you recognize these muscles, tighten them when *not* going to the bathroom, hold for a few seconds, and then relax. Do this tightening both quickly and slowly, but make sure not to hold your breath or tighten your abdomen. Kegels can be done up to one hundred times a day.

pelvic ring than men. We are built for childbirth. However, throughout the course of pregnancy the pelvic organs move up and they tend to become squashed from the enlarged uterus. The more space you can create, the more prana and blood can flow freely to your organs and to the baby. Poses that increase mobility in the hip and pelvic joints while strengthening and stretching the pelvic floor and perineal area are invaluable. Practicing this sequence regularly can facilitate greater comfort as pregnancy progresses, and possibly an easier childbirth.

This sequence uses some poses you learned in month four (see chapter 10).

1. CAKRAVAKASANA (RUDDY GOOSE POSE)

See page 112.

2. ADHO MUKHA SHVANASANA
   (DOWNWARD FACING DOG POSE)

See page 113.

3. TADASANA (MOUNTAIN POSE)

See page 109.

4. PARSHVA KONASANA (SIDE ANGLE POSE)

See page 112.

5. SQUATTING POSE

This pose is an adaptation of a pose known in various yoga traditions as Malasana (Garland Pose) and Utkatasana (Fierce Pose).

- Begin in Tadasana. If you would like more support, stand with your back against a wall.
- Widen your legs a couple feet and rotate your feet externally.
- Inhale, lengthen your spine, and sweep your arms up over your head.
- Exhale, bend your knees, and lower yourself into a squatting position. Lower your arms into a prayer position in front of your chest.

- Keep your feet and heels flat on the ground. If you are unable to do this pose with your heels firmly on the floor, fold a blanket and place it under your heels for extra support and stability. You can also lower your buttocks onto anything firm, such as yoga blocks or a rolled up blanket, if you feel uncomfortable in the squat and need more height in the pose.
- Lift and open the chest.
- Place your hands on your belly and send loving thoughts to your baby.
- Stay in your squat for three to twelve breaths. Do a few Kegels while in this pose. (See "Kegel Exercises," page 122.)
- When you are ready to come out of the pose, press your feet into the floor and use the strength of your legs or support of the wall to come up and out of the pose.

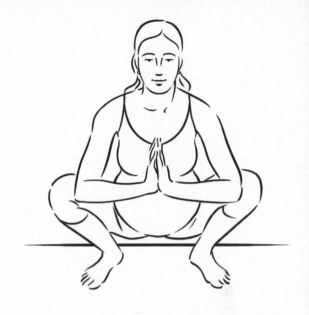

figure 12 **Squatting Pose**

6. PRASARITA PADOTTANASANA (EXTENDED LEG STRETCH)

See page 111.

7. BADDHA KONASANA (BOUND ANGLE POSE)

- Sit on your buttocks. If you are uncomfortable on the floor, elevate yourself by placing a folded blanket or two under your buttocks. Extend your legs out in front of you.
- Bring the soles of your feet together, and pull them close to your body. Open your knees wide and relax them toward the floor.
- Hold your ankles, or interlace your fingers and grasp under your feet.
- Inhale, lift your chest, and lengthen your crown toward the sky as you use your leg muscles to move your knees toward the floor. Avoid bending forward over your feet.
- Exhale and bring your knees up, still holding on to your feet or ankles as you do.

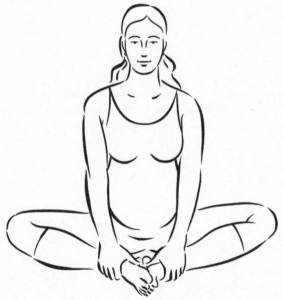

figure 13 **Baddha Konasana** (Bound Angle Pose)

- Move your legs up and down gently a few times, linking the movement to your breath. Then bring your knees toward the floor again, close your eyes, and stay for at least five breaths.
- Breathe into your inner legs, sacral area, and lower back. Keep your chest lifted and bring your shoulder blades toward each other. Keep your belly relaxed and your awareness on your breath.
- When you feel complete and are ready to come out of the pose, gently stretch your legs out in front of you, and then slowly move onto the next pose.

8. SHAVASANA
See page 115. ◈

BREATHING PRACTICE
Shitali Pranayama with Ujjayi Exhale and Counting

In this practice you will refine the practice from last month (shitali pranayama with ujjayi) with an added element of focus by counting your breaths. Begin with inhaling in a shitali mouth position and exhaling in ujjayi. While you are doing this, you can count the number of seconds in each inhalation and exhalation. Counting is solely for focus and variety. Do not try to do anything more than counting your breaths. It is important never to push your breath to the maximum; just stay with what is comfortable.

- Sit in a comfortable position. You can sit cross-legged on the floor, on a cushion in Sukhasana, or in a chair with your feet on the floor.
- Let the breath straighten the spine.
- Make an *O* shape with your mouth and curl your tongue inward. If you are not able to curl your tongue, simply place the tip of your tongue behind your two front teeth.
- Inhale air over your tongue as you slowly and gently lift your chin.
- When you finish, close your mouth; exhale through your nose as you direct the breath slowly across the back of your throat. This should create an ocean sound like waves crashing on the shore. Lower your head back to a neutral position while exhaling.

- Practice this technique for a few minutes. Then begin silently counting the number of seconds in your inhalation. For example, you may count slowly to three to reach the end of your inhalation.
- As you exhale, count the number of seconds in your exhalation.
- Continue counting for both the inhalation and exhalation for a total of twelve breaths. You can count on the digits of your hand as explained on page 84.
- Return to your normal breath and sit for a few moments before getting up. ◗

MEDITATION PRACTICE

You Are the Perfect Mother for Your Baby

This meditation uses a simple affirmation to create a profound positive impact. You can bring the meaning of the words within by linking your breath with each affirmation.

- Sit in a comfortable position. If you prefer to lie down, at this stage of pregnancy you should lie on your side, and use pillows under your head and between your legs. Let your breath be natural.
- Close your eyes. Take a few deep breaths to settle into your body. Feel your shoulders relax. Feel your jaw relax.
- Silently say the affirmation, "I am the perfect mother for my baby." Repeat the affirmation several times to yourself. Repeat it slowly.
- Let your words link to your breath with each inhale and each exhale: Inhaling—long and smooth breaths—"I am the perfect mother for my baby." And exhaling—long and smooth breaths—"I am the perfect mother for my baby."
- Feel the affirmation in your body, feel it in your bones, feel it in your heart, feel it with your breath, and feel it in your mind.
- Now place your hands on your belly. Continue saying the affirmation, linking it to your breath: Inhaling—long and smooth breaths—"I am the perfect mother for my baby." And exhaling— long and smooth breaths—"I am the perfect mother for my baby."
- Stay in this quiet state for a few more moments, repeating the affirmation to yourself with every in-breath and every out-breath.
- Open your eyes and sit quietly for a few moments before getting up. ◗

Sound Practice
Ma

The word *ma* means "mother" in many cultures around the world. The word *measure* comes from the Sanskrit root *ma,* and a mother is the one who is constantly measuring and assessing what is around her.

This simple practice uses the primary sound, *ma,* on different notes. Try to open your mouth wide and feel the sounds in your body as you honor your journey as a mother.

- Sit in a comfortable position.
- For each of the following phrases, take a natural breath in, then exhale, reciting one line per exhale:

Ma Ma Ma

Ma Ma Ma Ma

Ma Ma Ma Ma Ma

Ma Ma Ma

Ma Ma Ma Ma

Ma Ma Ma Ma Ma

- When finished, sit quietly for a few moments before getting up.

Month Six

SUPPORT

Stay with friends who support you in these. Talk with them about sacred texts,
and how you are doing, and how they are doing, and keep your practices together.
RUMI

Surrounding yourself with women who inspire, uplift, and support you is vital, particularly during pregnancy. The old and wise tenet of "keeping good company" has a special significance now. Referring back to chapter 4, "Harmonious Lifestyle," you may remember the importance of surrounding yourself with as much positivity as possible in order to bring that quality to your baby.

The inherent vulnerability of pregnancy makes it especially important for you to feel supported on various levels. You may feel sustained by a women's circle or by a girl's night out. Use your pregnancy as an opportunity, or even an excuse, to spend time with special women, which can deeply nourish your femininity and provide a special element of support only possible from other women.

The sixth month of pregnancy is an excellent time to begin thinking about having someone to support your labor, which can be long and intense. Continuous support during labor has been clinically proven to result in shorter labors with fewer complications, decreased need for medical intervention, and reduced negative feelings about one's childbirth experience. Furthermore, research demonstrates that parents who receive support feel more secure, have increased self-confidence, and are more successful in adapting to their changing family; supported moms have greater success with breastfeeding, and experience less postpartum depression.

You may choose to hire a doula or have a dear friend, sister, or mother support your labor. The most important aspect is your comfort level. Choose someone who will help you to feel at ease, inspire confidence, and deeply support your most intense and intimate moments. An experienced and skilled woman, preferably someone who has been through childbirth, is an excellent choice.

Sometimes women feel they *should* invite their mother or sister to be at their birth. But remember, your childbirth experience is about *your* wishes and not about others and what they want. Lots of women would love to be at a birth, but who attends is ultimately your and your partner's decision. Whomever you choose should be okay with whatever you do, even if you decide at the end that you do not want them present at the birth.

A doula can be an anchor during the birth, as well as toward the end of your pregnancy and during postpartum. The word *doula* originates from an ancient Greek word meaning "a woman who serves." Doula now refers to a trained and experienced woman who provides continuous physical, emotional, and informational support to a mother before, during, and just after birth, or someone who provides emotional and practical support during the postpartum period.

The value of a doula cannot be underestimated. She can discuss your fears about birth and motherhood, answer your questions, and be available for overall support. She may also be able to help you release previous traumatic birth experiences before you give birth again. And she can often be more objective than a close family member or friend, which can be advantageous.

You may need to interview several doulas with your partner. It is important that *both* of you feel comfortable with her. See the resources section for information on how to find a doula.

When I was pregnant with my daughter, I only wanted my husband and midwife present at the birth. I wanted the privacy and intimacy to be shared only with them. After my labor did not progress, I realized there was a missing element of support that could have helped me to have a more positive, natural birth experience. In my second pregnancy, I was certain I wanted a doula and chose a wonderful woman named Autumn, whose experience and nurturing hands and heart were astounding. As the pregnancy progressed, I grew to feel very close to Autumn. Her extraordinary, solid presence at my son's birth facilitated the natural birth I had envisioned.

Birth Vision

Many women enjoy writing down their visions for birth, which can be helpful for everyone supporting their labor. This is an opportunity for you, and perhaps your partner, to ponder ahead of time what you wish for labor. It is a vision and a hope. However, it is *essential* to be aware that many aspects of labor cannot be controlled and to be open-minded to whatever comes, including things that may be outside of your vision. Truly staying in the present moment and releasing expectations are perhaps the best birth visions!

When I was pregnant with my daughter, I held on very tightly to my birth vision. I didn't realize it at the time, but I was almost gripping to it. My birth experience turned out exactly the opposite of what I'd envisioned. I didn't end up giving birth under candlelight in a tub in our sacred bedroom. Instead, I was induced, numbed, and confined to a hospital bed.

Thankfully, I was a little wiser the second time around. I had my vision but was completely *not* attached to it, and stayed open to the true magic and mystery of birth. Through a more open-minded vision, I became empowered to birth my son naturally, quickly, and smoothly.

You can begin to think about:

- Who would you like to be present as you give birth?
- How would you like the atmosphere to be? For example, would you like dim lights or music?
- What labor props (such as a birthing ball or a stool) would you like available?
- How would you like interventions to be handled, if necessary?
- What are your wishes for immediately after the baby comes? For example, would you like the baby placed on your chest if possible, before the baby is washed? What would you like to do with the placenta?

Dharma

I have discussed the word *dharma* a few other places in this book already. Dharma means "duty, responsibility, and purpose," which includes work and career, but also encompasses much more. Dharma comes from the Sanskrit root meaning "to support." It is said that if you support dharma, it will support you and your role in life. It is almost like a force that prevents something from falling down and that can pick up what has fallen.

We have many dharmas throughout our lifetime—dharmas to our families, to our jobs, to our education, to our society, and to our other relationships. Often, it is not clear what one's dharma is. Action is needed to understand and discover your dharmas. You cannot sit around and ponder; it is through action, exploration, and observation that they are revealed.

It is also important to be cognizant of your dharmas at different points in life, because they will change. Right now, you have a dharma to your pregnancy. Your primary responsibility is to take care of yourself, perhaps like never before, and the baby growing in your belly. But life is often not simple, and you may have conflicting dharmas. At the same time as you have a dharma to your pregnancy, you may also have a dharma to your family, to your partner, and to your career. If you had a significant professional life before pregnancy, it may be difficult to shift gears to make your health and that of your growing baby the highest priority. You may need to adjust your diet to incorporate important prenatal nutrients or take five-minute breaks from sitting at your desk to stretch and breathe. Staying up late and eating on the run may wreak havoc on different levels of your system that were not apparent before your pregnancy. The guidance in this book supports your dharma of pregnancy.

JOURNALING EXERCISE

Exploring Your Dharmas and Support

Prioritizing your goals, with your dharmas as a reference point, is immensely helpful. In today's world it is easy to lose the idea of responsibility or dharma. Ask yourself:

- What are my different responsibilities and duties? To what and to whom?
- How can I fulfill them?
- Do I feel supported in my dharmas? How?

Take a few minutes and jot down your ideas.

This is also an appropriate time in your pregnancy to think about support for you and your family after the baby arrives. Ask yourself: Ideally, what support would I like? Someone to hold the baby while I take a shower or a nap? Help with meals? Playdates for my older children? Then take the next step and begin exploring practical means of getting the support you will need after the baby comes. ◗

ASANA PRACTICE
Supported Restorative Poses

Supported restorative poses feel heavenly in pregnancy. A restorative practice is an opportunity to let the body deeply rest, unwind, and release. These poses also promote a feeling of receptivity in the body. This sequence is excellent for the later afternoon, or before dinner or bedtime. Hopefully, you will feel renewed, calm, and relaxed after doing it.

For many of these poses, have on hand several blankets, a yoga bolster, and/or a couple of yoga blocks (if you have them).

1. CAKRAVAKASANA (RUDDY GOOSE POSE)
See page 112.

2. BALASANA (CHILD'S POSE)

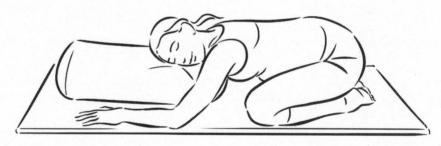

- Sit on your bent knees, which are wide apart.
- Bring your forehead toward the floor and let it rest on a bolster, pillow, or block. Stretch your arms in front of you.

figure 14 **Balasana** (Child's Pose)

- Your buttocks are toward your heels. You may need to lift your buttocks higher as your pregnancy progresses.
- Rest in the pose for a few minutes, as long as it's comfortable. Feel your pelvic canal widening and the mobility of your pelvic joints increasing, while your lower back, sacrum, and hips relax.
- When you're ready to come out of the pose, push your hands into the floor and use the strength of your arms to push up your torso.

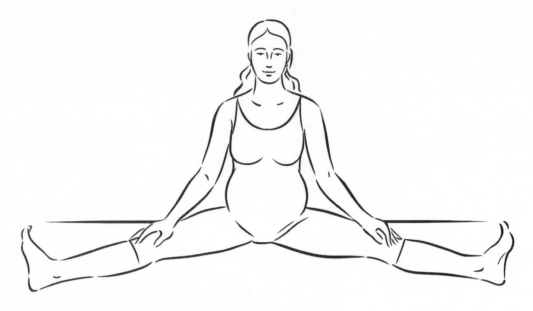

figure 15 **Upavishta Konasana** (Wide Angle Pose)

3. UPAVISHTA KONASANA
(WIDE ANGLE POSE)

- Sit directly on the floor, or elevate your buttocks by sitting on a folded blanket, with your legs straight in front of you. Then spread your legs wide.
- Flex your feet and engage your leg muscles by pressing the backs of your legs down.
- Inhale as you lengthen the spine upward and lift your arms by your ears.
- Exhale, lower your arms, and gently walk your hands in front of you.
- Inhale and bring your torso back up.
- Repeat three times.
- The third time you walk your hands forward, rest your head and arms on a bolster for several breaths.
- When you are ready to come out of the pose, press your hands into the floor and use the strength of your arms to bring yourself back to the starting position.

4. CAKRAVAKASANA
(RUDDY GOOSE POSE)

- Repeat Cakravakasana as a counterpose.

5. SUPTA BADDHA KONASANA (RECLINING BOUND ANGLE POSE)

- Sit on the floor with a bolster or a few rolled up blankets placed two to four inches behind your pelvis, parallel to your spine. Your legs are straight out in front of you.
- Bend your knees so you can bring the soles of your feet together, close to your body. Place extra rolled up blankets under your knees for support, if needed.
- Recline back onto the bolster or blankets, with your spine in the middle. Place a separate blanket under your head for support. Rest your arms by your side, palms facing up.
- Take a couple natural breaths and let your body feel open and relaxed.
- Now sweep your outstretched arms in front of you and move your hands up over your head. Then sweep your arms back down by your side, as if you are making a snow angel. Do this arm movement several times.
- Relax your arms by your sides again, with your palms facing up and elbows relaxed.
- Stay in the pose for several long and smooth breaths. You may enjoy staying in this pose for five minutes, if time allows.
- When you are ready to come out of the pose, bring your knees together and place the soles of your feet flat on the floor. Slowly roll to the right side, and then raise yourself into a sitting position before getting up off the floor.

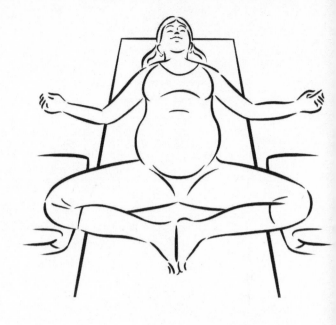

figure 16 **Supta Baddha Konasana** (Reclining Bound Angle Pose)

6. SHAVASANA (CORPSE POSE)

See page 115.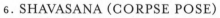

BREATHING PRACTICE

Nadi Shodhana Pranayama

Nadi means "channel," and *shodhana* means "cleaning or purifying." Nadi shodhana, or alternate-nostril breathing, is thought to purify the subtle channels within the body so prana (breath or life force) flows more freely and smoothly. This technique is thought to reduce stress and anxiety while promoting relaxation and a lowered heart rate. Traditionally, nadi shodhana includes fixed breathing ratios and retention of the breath, which are strong practices not appropriate in pregnancy. And traditionally, this practice is done using the right hand, but feel free to use your left if that is more comfortable.

- Sit in a comfortable position—cross-legged on the floor, on a cushion in Sukhasana, or seated in a chair.
- Take a deep breath and let your breath lengthen your spine as you sit up tall.
- Bring your right hand to your nose and gently close your right nostril with your thumb. Calmly and smoothly inhale through your left nostril, and then close your left nostril with your ring and little fingers. Move your right thumb to open your right nostril. Slowly exhale through your right nostril.
- Keep the right nostril open, slowly inhale, and then close it with your thumb. Open the left nostril and exhale slowly. This is one cycle.
- Repeat this cycle twelve times, counting the cycles on the inner digits of your hand, as explained on page 84.
- When you are finished, release your hand to your lap and breathe naturally for a few breaths before getting up. ◗

MEDITATION PRACTICE

Support from the Mountains

Mountains have always been symbols of great power, incredible energy, and awesome beauty. They seem to possess an invincible force of strength. With its images of mountains, this meditation can help you feel supported in your life. As you visualize the mountains, their positive qualities and their forces can come to you.

If you have a clear image of a specific mountain or mountain chain in your mind, please use that for this meditation. Or to inspire your vision, you may wish to find a picture from a magazine, a photo album, or the Internet. Place the image in front of you before you begin.

- Sit in a comfortable position.
- Look at your picture and then close your eyes.
- Take several slow, full breaths to bring your awareness to your life force—your breath, your prana.
- Visualize a majestic mountain or mountain chain.
- Notice that your seated posture resembles a mountain itself, with a broad base tapering to a summit at the top of your head.
- Visualize yourself *as* the mountain—stable, solid, and still— bringing in these qualities of support from Mother Nature.
- Let each breath connect you back to your vision and help you to take in the positive qualities of your mountain: stability, strength, and confidence.
- When you feel complete, gradually open your eyes and sit quietly for a few moments before getting up. ◗

SOUND PRACTICE
Asato Ma

"Asato Ma" is a popular chant about moving toward goodness and truth-fulness. This chant says, "Lead me from the unreal to real, lead me from darkness to light, lead me from what is impermanent to what is eternal." Let this chant support you in becoming a more conscious woman, mother, partner, and friend.

- Begin by sitting comfortably. You can sit cross-legged on the floor, on a cushion in Sukhasana, or in a chair.
- For each of the following phrases, take a natural breath in, then exhale, reciting one line per exhale:

Asato ma (asah-tow maa)
Sadgamaya (sad-gah-mah-yah)
Tamaso ma (tah-mah-so maa)
Jyotir gamaya (jyo-teer gah-mah-yah)
Mrtyorma (mrit-yor-maa)
Amritam gamaya (amritahm gah-mah-yah)
Asato ma sadgamaya
Tamaso ma jyotirgamaya
Mrtyorma amritam gamaya

• When finished, sit quietly for a few moments before getting up. ◗

The Third Trimester

Observe how endings become beginnings.
Lao Tzu

The final leg of your journey has arrived. Ten lunar months of pregnancy, roughly equal to nine solar months, is almost a full cycle around the sun, giving you the opportunity to weather nearly every season. You are undoubtedly a stronger woman from it. I've always felt that the duration of pregnancy is the perfect amount of time to prepare for the rigors and rewards of motherhood.

Many women feel that they cannot possibly become any larger at this point, but both mama and baby need to keep growing throughout the course of this trimester. Staying positive is key now and through the birth, because you will be meeting your new little one soon!

What's Happening in Your Body?

The following sections present general information on your baby's growth and development and typical physical and emotional changes during pregnancy. This is not an exhaustive list and there are always variations within the normal range. Every woman's experience of pregnancy is unique, whether it is your first or your fifth. Also, please keep in mind that there is an immeasurable element of mystery during pregnancy that continually creates new experiences.

The fetus is continuously gaining weight, typically entering the seventh month around two and a half pounds and becoming six to nine pounds at birth. The lungs, digestive system, and heat control systems are still developing. By twenty-nine weeks your baby's bones are fully developed, even though they are soft and pliable. The brain continues to develop rapidly.

By thirty-six weeks your baby's reflexes are coordinated so she can blink, close her eyes, turn her head, grasp firmly, smile, frown, and yawn. She can respond to sounds, light, and touch through the abdominal wall. You may notice her movements more clearly now as the close quarters in your uterus can make her stretches and rolls more obvious. Some babies can be very active, especially male babies. I remember feeling my son's kicks quite strongly. Toward the end of my pregnancy, my husband and I watched my tummy as our little boy's hand or foot protruded from my skin and moved across my entire belly. It was wild to see!

After thirty-seven weeks your baby is considered full term. Her vital organs are ready to function on their own. Hopefully, your little one will hang out inside for a few more weeks to get stronger and healthier before life outside the womb begins.

TYPICAL PHYSICAL CHANGES

Increased weight gain. By the time your due date approaches you may be twenty to thirty-five pounds heavier than before your pregnancy. Your baby accounts for some of the weight gain. The placenta, amniotic fluid, larger breasts and uterus, extra fat stores, and increased blood and fluid volume account for the rest.

Continued breast growth. The breasts are much fuller and larger at this point, often with two pounds of extra tissue. They may leak colostrum, a yellowish, liquid substance that will nourish your baby during the first few days of life.

Shortness of breath. The uterus expands beneath the diaphragm and can place pressure on your lungs. Your lungs are also processing more air than they did before your pregnancy, which allows your blood to carry more oxygen to your placenta and baby. This can cause you to breathe slightly faster and experience shortness of breath.

Swelling. The growing uterus puts pressure on the veins that return blood from the feet and legs, creating swollen feet and ankles.

Frequent urination. Many moms-to-be feel pressure on their bladder as the baby moves deeper into the pelvis, causing more frequent urination. This extra pressure may cause you to leak urine, especially when you laugh, cough, or sneeze.

Braxton-Hicks contractions. These are weak, irregular, unpredictable contractions to prepare you for the real thing. Contact your prenatal care provider if your contractions are painful or regular.

Sore back. It's easy for your back to become sore as you adjust to the extra weight, the effects of hormones relaxing your muscles and ligaments, and perhaps an altered posture that can cause you to walk in a different way than you have previously.

Varicose veins and hemorrhoids. Varicose veins, blue or reddish lines beneath the surface of the skin, are basically swollen blood vessels that can appear or worsen during pregnancy. They primarily show up in the legs due to the increased blood volume, your growing uterus putting pressure on the pelvic veins, and the relaxation of the veins from pregnancy hormones. Varicose veins can also occur in your rectum as hemorrhoids.

Heartburn. The flap (lower esophageal sphincter) at the top of your stomach, which is usually closed to prevent digestive acids from splashing into the esophagus, relaxes from pregnancy hormones and allows the acids to go back up, creating heartburn. Since the uterus has taken up most of your abdominal cavity, it pushes your stomach up and creates heartburn as well.

TYPICAL EMOTIONAL CHANGES

The third trimester can be challenging, both physically and emotionally. You may feel physically uncomfortable because of your baby's size and position. In the third trimesters of my own pregnancies, I felt like an over-ripe peach dangling from a tree: so full and just waiting to burst. You may be ready to move beyond pregnancy and onto the next stage of your life. Staying in the present moment and remaining optimistic are essential for being able to enjoy the end of your pregnancy.

Try not to compare your body to those of other pregnant women, as all women carry their babies differently. Pregnant bellies can be high, low, big, small, wide or compact. It all depends on your body's structure, your weight gain, and your baby's size and position.

At the end of pregnancy, women often feel spacey and find it hard to focus on work and details. Use this as an opportunity to let go of some responsibilities (if possible), to daydream, and to enjoy doing simple things. Envision carrying your baby in your arms. Sit under a tree and ponder baby names, or partake in other creative, dreamy activities.

Many women experience mixed emotions in the third trimester: excitement, anxiety, bliss, and feeling overwhelmed are a few. You may wonder how you will manage family, work, personal time, adjusting to motherhood, and the changes in your relationships, especially if you already have one or more children. Talking to other mothers can shed light on the joys and challenges of expanding your family and help you feel more prepared for motherhood.

You may also be curious about what the birth will be like, if you will be able to handle the pain, and if you will have the right support. Remember that you have all the strength inside yourself to birth your baby, and babies come into the world a multitude of ways. The ultimate goal is a healthy mom and healthy baby. There are no right or wrong ways to give birth.

Fear, both your own and your partner's, may be more pronounced in the third trimester. The thought of a baby coming can make some partners feel that they are not ready for parenthood and can bring up issues like not wanting to repeat the mistakes of their parents. Men often handle third trimester emotions differently than women. I remember feeling that my husband was not as excited as I was in the last few months. This was completely untrue, and I came to see that his way of expressing his excitement and anticipation was different than mine. He wasn't doting over adorable, tiny newborn clothing like I was, but enjoyed assembling the birthing tub, car seat, and changing table. He needed to use his hands to tangibly create something for our baby. That process helped him emotionally to become ready for our new life as parents.

14

Month Seven

OPENING THE HEART

Compassion is the very essence of an open heart and must be cultivated throughout our journey.
THE DALAI LAMA

According to Ayurveda, the heart is the seat of prana, ojas, and the center of love and compassion. It is the place in the spiritual body where feminine and masculine energies meet. These energies come together in intimate, divine love that is pure, boundless, and unconditional. This love has nothing to do with sex.

In the heart resides the inner aspect of yourself that is unchanging—your spirit, called *purusha*, and considered your inner light of awareness. This divine light emanates love and compassion. Being loving, open-hearted, and compassionate is a state of mind that you can direct toward others, toward yourself, and toward your baby. The baby will pick up feelings of love and compassion in the womb and carry them for the rest of his life. The intimacy between a mother and her baby begins with an open heart.

If feeling compassionate is a challenge for you, then this is an opportunity to cultivate more for yourself. Beginning today, send yourself the message that you love every ounce of who you are. Cultivating compassion for others begins with listening honestly, forgiving freely, being generous, and emanating lovingkindness. You may find that compassion for others grows naturally from having compassion for yourself.

When you are carrying a baby in your belly, your heart may feel extra sensitive and vulnerable. The heart is where we feel hurt, grief, and rejection. The journey into the heart can be difficult, since this is where we confront these feelings and are called to move through and beyond them. Women's hearts seem to be more delicate than their male counterparts, especially in pregnancy. You may find yourself randomly crying, perhaps from a sappy commercial on TV or something more profound that pulls on your heartstrings. Know that these experiences are perfectly natural as you move through the practices for this month.

Let this time in your pregnancy be an excuse to pick or buy yourself a bouquet of flowers. Choose beautiful colors and lovely aromas that delight your heart and bring happiness to you.

Heart-Opening Tea

Lemon balm, one of the main ingredients in this tea, is known as the "gladdening herb" as its pleasant fragrance can instantly lift your spirits and open your heart, among many other benefits.

To make a pot of heart-opening tea, place 1 heaping teaspoon each of lemon balm, lemon verbena, and linden flowers, ½ teaspoon each of hibiscus flowers and rosehips, and a few rose petals. Cover with 2 cups of boiling water and infuse for 10–15 minutes. Strain and sweeten with 1 teaspoon of honey.

Savor the warmth, aroma, and sweetness, either alone or with your partner or close friend.

Exploring Your Changing Relationship

Sometimes partners in relationship seem to be from different planets, especially regarding sexuality. Handling different libidos in pregnancy can be challenging for many couples. Some women feel incredibly sexy with a superstrong libido. Others feel too full of baby and have no interest in sex. And a woman's feelings about sex can change from month to month.

If one partner is having a difficult time cooling down their fire, they can find other ways to release their energy, like physical activity. It is vital for your relationship to explore intimacy without intercourse, to build a foundation of respect and trust for each other.

Classical Ayurvedic texts do not encourage sex during pregnancy; however, this guidance is set in a historical, socio-religious context where sex was primarily for procreation. Modern science does not restrict sex during a normal pregnancy with no complications. Many couples feel that making love during pregnancy helps to keep their blood and energy circulating and has a releasing and opening effect on the body. If you and your partner are on the same page, the greatest challenge may be finding positions that are enjoyable and comfortable for both of you.

Frequently, couples wonder how lovemaking and orgasms affect the baby. You may notice that the baby seems very quiet or inactive after you and your partner make love. Perhaps the rhythmic movements lull him to sleep. You may also notice that your baby is much more active afterward. Both are normal responses. The baby isn't aware of sexual situations as such, but he can feel his mother's physical motions, as well as warm, positive emotions.

Unless your healthcare provider tells you to cool it, there is no reason not to. You can enjoy making love and having orgasms right up until delivery, and passionate lovemaking may even help your body move into labor more quickly.

JOURNALING EXERCISE
Exploring Intimacy with Your Partner

Do this exercise with your partner, as an opening for a conversation and an opportunity to become closer.

Write in your journals individually. Each of you ask yourself:

- How has our intimacy changed during the pregnancy?
- What do I enjoy?
- What is a challenge?
- What, if anything, do I wish were different?

Then take turns sharing what you wrote. Listen from your heart. Do not interrupt each other.

Let this exercise lead into the following practice. ◊

FUN PRACTICE
Creative Intimacy

Ultimately, intimacy is about connection, and it can happen with or without intercourse. Use this stage of your pregnancy as an occasion to be creative and share intimacy and love with your partner in new ways. Some ideas are:

- taking a bath together
- exchanging a foot or full-body massage
- making music or singing together
- sharing a candlelight dinner
- leaving love notes for each other
- meditating or praying together

If you are a single mother, you may enjoy sharing these or similar activities with a close friend. ◖

Opening the Heart

Opening the heart energetically comes more easily when there are few obstructions in the physical body. The weight of new breast tissue can feel heavy and cause the chest to collapse forward, which subsequently places strain on the back and neck. The poses in this practice sequence help to open up the heart area, to create a sense of lightness, openness, and freedom.

In all these poses, pay extra attention to the heart, chest, and lung area. Allow your inhalation to move the prana into the lungs; feel the expansion of the intercostal muscles as the heart space opens. Observe how you feel before and after the practice.

1. TADASANA (MOUNTAIN POSE)
See page 109.

2. VIRABHADRASANA (WARRIOR POSE)
See page 110.

3. SQUATTING POSE
See page 122. *Skip this pose if you are thirty-four weeks or more along and your baby is in a breech position.*

4. TRIKONASANA (TRIANGLE POSE)

- Begin in Tadasana.
- Step your feet three to four feet apart, sideways.
- Turn your left toes inward about forty-five degrees and your right leg outward ninety degrees. Your heels should be in line with one another.
- Inhale and lift your arms to shoulder level.
- Exhale and laterally bend your torso to the right as far as comfortable.
- Place your right hand somewhere on your right leg, thigh, calf, or foot. You can also place your hand on a yoga block or a chair.
- Look up at your left hand, which is pointing toward the sky.
- Breathe slowly and stay in the posture for three to four breaths.
- Rotate your head to look toward the floor. Hold this position for another two breaths.
- Inhale and use the strength of your upper body to bring yourself back to the starting position.
- Turn your feet in the opposite direction and repeat on the other side.
- Step your legs together when finished.

5. PRASARITA PADOTTANASANA (EXPANDED LEG STRETCH)

See page 111.

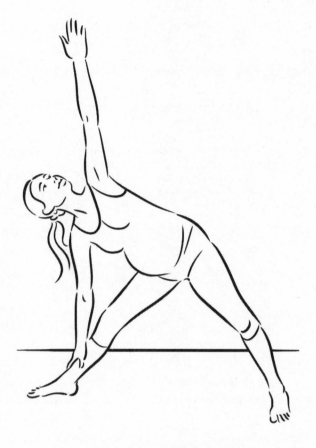

figure 17 **Trikonasana** (Triangle Pose)

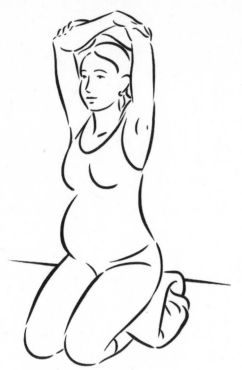

figure 18 **Virasana with Arm Movements** (Hero Pose)

6. VIRASANA WITH ARM MOVEMENTS (HERO POSE)

- Sit on your knees with a few blankets stacked between your heels and your buttocks.
- Exhale, interlace your fingers, and flip your palms so that they're facing away from you. Straighten your elbows, extending your arms in front of you.
- Inhale and lift your outstretched arms above your head, keeping your arms in line with your ears.
- Exhale and bend your elbows to bring your clasped hands behind your head.
- Inhale and lift your outstretched arms back above your head, keeping your arms in line with your ears.
- Exhale and lower your arms in front of you, to the level of your breasts, keeping your fingers interlaced, palms facing away from you, elbows bent.
- Inhale and lift your outstretched arms above your head, keeping your arms in line with your ears. Grasp each elbow with the opposite hand.
- Stay in this position for three to four long, smooth breaths.
- Release your hands and arms to your sides.
- Repeat the pose by interlacing your fingers the opposite way and doing the entire series of arm movements again.

7. CAKRAVAKASANA (RUDDY GOOSE POSE)
See page 112.

8. SHAVASANA (CORPSE POSE)
See page 115. ◗

BREATHING PRACTICE
Shitali with Alternate-Nostril Pranayama

This practice combines two breathing practices from previous months. You will inhale in a shitali mouth position and exhale using nadi shodhana alternate-nostril breathing. These practices enable you to more effectively regulate the length of your exhalation and challenge your mental focus.

- Sit in a comfortable position. You can sit cross-legged on the floor, on a cushion in Sukhasana, or in a chair.
- Breathe naturally for a few moments. Let your breath straighten your spine.
- Make an O shape with your mouth and curl your tongue if you are able. If you are not able to curl your tongue, simply place the tip of your tongue behind your two front teeth.
- Inhale air over your tongue as you slowly and gently lift your chin. You will feel the cold air coming into your mouth. It is as if your curled tongue were a straw, and you're sucking the air in through it.
- When you finish, close your mouth, bring your right hand to your nose, and gently close your right nostril with your thumb. Slowly exhale through your left nostril as you bring your chin back to neutral.
- Return your hand to your lap.
- Inhale again in shitali mouth position, raising your chin. Close your mouth, bring your right hand to your nose, and gently close your left nostril with your pinky and ring finger. Slowly exhale through your right nostril as you bring your chin back to neutral.
- Return your hand to your lap. You have completed one breath cycle.
- Repeat this exercise twelve times, once again counting on the inner digits of your hand.
- When finished, return to your natural breath and sit for a few moments before getting up. ◗

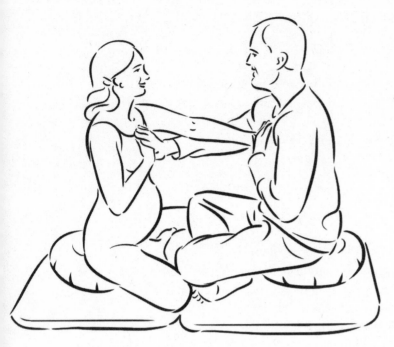

MEDITATION PRACTICE

Partner Meditation, Sending Love

This practice, as the name suggests, is to be done with someone else. It can be either with your partner or a close friend.

- Sit in a comfortable position, and place your spine against your partner's spine. If sitting on the floor isn't comfortable for you or your partner, you can use backless stools or other objects that allow you to sit with your spines touching.
- Close your eyes and take a few full and calm breaths to settle in. Don't try to regulate your breath—just let it be relaxed.

figure 19 **Partner Meditation** Sending Love

- Feel your partner's breath moving in their body against yours.
- Feel your heart center opening, and visualize pouring love from your heart right into your partner's heart. Send them an abundance of loving energy.
- As you inhale, receive the love your partner is sending you. As you exhale, send love to your partner. Continue this exchange for several breaths.
- Now turn toward your partner. Sit so you are facing each other.
- Place one hand on your own heart and the other hand on your partner's heart. Have them do the same, placing their hands on top of yours (see figure 19).
- Close your eyes and breathe together, feeling the rise and fall of both of your chests and bellies.
- Send loving energy and lovingkindness toward each other.
- Inhale and receive the love your partner is sending. Exhale and send love to your partner. See love infusing every cell of their body.
- Now both of you place all four hands on your belly. Close your eyes.

- Inhale and imagine all your love and positive energy joining together. Exhale and send it all to your baby. Breathe together, with all four hands on your belly, for several breaths.
- When you both feel complete, open your eyes, look softly into each other's eyes, and hug each other. ◗

SOUND PRACTICE

Hridayam Mayi

This sound practice is taken from a longer chant called "Laghunyasa." This chant asks the various elements of nature to nourish different aspects of the human system. The lines you will be reciting translate to: "The heart is in me. I am in the divine essence. The divine essence is everywhere."

- Sit in a comfortable position. You can sit cross-legged on the floor, on a cushion in Sukhasana, or in a chair.
- Let the breath lengthen the spine.
- For each of the following phrases, take a natural breath in, then exhale, reciting one line per exhale.

Hridayam (hrid-ah-yum)

Mayi (mah-yee)

Hridayam Mayi (hrid-ay-yum mah-yee)

Aham (ah-hum)

Amrite (ahm-ri-tay-ay)

Aham Amrite (ah-hum ahm-ri-tay-ay)

Amritam (ahm-ri-tum)

Brahmani (brahm-huh-nee)

Amritam Brahmani (ahm-ri-tum brahm-huh-nee)

Hridayam Mayi

Aham Amrite

Amritam Brahmani

- Now place your hands on top of each other on your heart. Inhale through your nose with your mouth closed. As you exhale, recite "Hridayam Mayi."

- As you inhale again, slowly move your hands off your chest and open your arms as wide as you can. As you exhale, recite "Aham Amrite."
- Inhale and bring your hands back onto your heart. As you exhale, recite "Amritam Brahmani."
- Do the last three steps, with the gestures, two more times.
- When finished, sit quietly for a few moments before getting up. ◉

15

Month Eight

BALANCE AND BLESSING

May the warm winds of heaven blow softly upon your house.
May the Great Spirit bless all who enter there.
May your moccasins make happy tracks in many snows,
and may the rainbow always touch your shoulder.
CHEROKEE PRAYER BLESSING

A huge wave of anxiety swept over me in the eighth month of my first pregnancy. I was worried that I wouldn't know what to do in labor, and I would forget everything I had been practicing. And even though I was overjoyed to become a mother, I also felt nervous about how much my life would change. I wondered if I could still travel freely, and if I would feel satisfied staying home with the baby for a year.

Nervousness and anxiety, characteristic emotions of imbalanced Vata dosha, are natural and understandable, especially during pregnancy. To create more harmony for myself, I followed a basic Vata-reducing program of eating warming, well-cooked, and spiced foods. I got plenty of rest and spent several days a week swimming and massaging warm sesame oil all over my very pregnant body. My teacher and mentor taught me a chant to invoke divine qualities in my growing baby. Through chanting slowly and

151

calmly, I began to feel very relaxed in my body and mind. I practiced daily an asana called Supta Baddha Konasana (explained on page 133), extending the exhalations to relax my nervous system, while my body softened and I visualized a smooth labor. Within a few weeks, my anxiety diminished significantly, and I felt more grounded and prepared for what lay ahead.

The month finished with a birth blessing ceremony guided by my friend Nina. She organized a circle of my closest women friends to gather and prepare me for my new journey. All the women brought candles, a blessing, and part of a meal to share. Nina began the ceremony, smudging everyone with sage and waving an eagle feather to energetically clear the space. Each woman came up to me, one by one, and gave me a blessing for the birth and my new life. We all shared a meal illuminated by candlelight. My heart felt blown open as I realized how special each relationship truly was. At the end of the ceremony, Nina organized a sign-up sheet for women to prepare home-cooked meals for me after the baby arrived. I left feeling deeply nurtured, inspired, and confident about the changes to come.

Instability of Ojas

"Ojas is the essence of the body responsible for strength, natural resistance and is considered essential for life," says the Ashtanga Hridayam, a classic Ayurvedic text. "It is said to be present in the heart. . . . Its presence in the fetus and mother produce strength and contentment, and its absence fatigue and anxiety."

I now see that the vacillation of my emotions during this eighth month was perhaps from an instability of ojas. Almost every classical Ayurvedic text talks about how ojas moves from the mother to the fetus and from the fetus to the mother in the eighth month. Because of this transfer, it is said that the mother and fetus alternately become happy and energetic when ojas is strong, then fatigued and anxious when ojas is weak. The instability of ojas makes it an unfavorable time to give birth, both for the mother and for the baby's health.

You may notice yourself feeling surges of energy coming and going, obviously or subtly. You may also not notice anything, which is completely fine. Either way, this month is an opportune time to replenish your ojas by following a diet and lifestyle appropriate to your constitution. If you have strayed from following a diet that is in harmony with your dosha, now is an ideal time to come back to it.

Ojas can be fortified by eating foods that build and nourish, and by doing wholesome, rejuvenating activities and yogic practices. You may notice that some foods and activities will have more noticeable and immediate effects on your energy and vitality, while others will take longer to kick in. Regardless of what you feel or notice, replenishing and supporting your ojas will help you to feel balanced, strong, and healthy through the end of your pregnancy and into postpartum.

Building Ojas

WITH FOODS	almonds and walnuts
	dates and figs
	honey (avoid raw honey in pregnancy)
	sesame seeds
	fresh fruits and fresh pressed juice
	saffron and cardamom
	fresh ghee, butter, and milk (particularly warm, spiced milk)
	fresh coconut
	whole grains, like wheat
	split mung beans
	root vegetables (like yams)
WITH NOURISHING ACTIVITIES	being in nature
	sleeping soundly
	spending time away from computers, telephones, and televisions
	performing oil self-massage daily
	taking a relaxing vacation
WITH YOGIC PRACTICES	meditation
	chanting
	certain breathing exercises outlined in this book
WITH HERBS	ayurvedic (tridoshic) herbal jelly called chyavanprash (safe in pregnancy if certified and tested organic)
	ashwagandha and shatavari (use under the guidance of an ayurvedic practitioner or herbalist, specializing in pregnancy)

JOURNALING EXERCISE

Blessings in Your Life

With all the signs around you that birth is imminent, and the inherent stress, anxiety, and excitement the end of your pregnancy brings, let this be an opportunity to focus on gratitude as a way to feel balanced. When you shift your thinking to highlight what is optimistic and encouraging in your life, no matter how small or large it may be, inner feelings of contentment arise. Acknowledging and reinforcing the positive gives less attention to the negative, which then weakens.

In chapter 2, under "Mind: Meditation," I discussed the idea of a bhavana, or intention. Bhavana can be specific to a yoga or meditation practice but can also be used in a larger context. You can have a bhavana for a conversation, for a project, or for a day, week, or month. Use this time to have a bhavana of gratitude, which can arise from this journaling exercise.

For this journaling exercise, write down at least ten blessings in your life. You can make a list or just write freestyle in your journal. Blessings come in all shapes and sizes. They can be anything from a friend offering to pick your child up from school so you can enjoy an afternoon nap, a feeling of gratitude for working part-time at the end of your pregnancy, to an awareness of the growing relationship with your partner. You can also make mental blessing lists while lying in bed or stuck in traffic—if that is easier for you—and write them down in your journal later. Try to do this exercise every day for one week. Once you notice how this exercise affects your overall mood, you may want to continue doing it for the rest of your pregnancy—and beyond. ◊

FUN PRACTICE

Hip Circles, Figure Eights, and Dancing

Moving your hips and dancing are fun practices that help increase circulation and energy while bringing a sense of lightness and joy to the body.

Put on your favorite music. Start with making hip circles, which are just circular motions with your hips, moving in both directions. Then move into making figure eights, again in both directions. Then move as you wish, open up, and dance if time and space allow. Close your eyes, tune inside, place your hands on your belly, and celebrate yourself.

But don't overdo it! I pulled all the muscles in my ribs, dancing at a wedding in my third trimester. I felt so open and free that I just danced, danced, and danced. I had such a great time that I didn't regret it, but I was very sore for about two weeks.

To spice things up and add a little free movement into your practice, you can also add hip circles and figure eights into your yoga practice when doing standing poses. ◗

Rituals and Blessings to Prepare for Birth and Motherhood

Our modern culture has become accustomed to preparing women for birth and motherhood in a material sense. Every woman will need clothes and blankets for her new child, and baby showers are a fun and wonderful time to receive such generosity.

On a deeper level, honoring pregnancy as a rite of passage helps a woman to prepare mentally, emotionally, and spiritually for the work of birthing and becoming a mother. This inevitably creates feelings of confidence, strength, and support for her new stage of life.

A ceremony to honor the mother-to-be and her sacred journey through pregnancy, in keeping with her personal belief system and involving important people in her life, can provide a deeply meaningful and transformational experience. Family traditions, birth blessings, rituals, and any kind of spiritual, religious, and/or creative practices or activities can be incorporated into the ceremony. The possibilities are endless. Here are some ideas:

Prayers, poems, and blessings written for the mother-to-be. Guests can also read appropriate prayers, poems, and blessing written by other writers. Each woman can hold a ball of yarn while reading her prayers or poems to the mother-to-be and pass it on. At the end, each woman cuts a piece of yarn to wear as a bracelet or anklet to remind her to hold the pregnant mama in her heart and mind until after the birth.

Candles and fires create a warm and sacred atmosphere. Each person can light a candle while she says her blessing.

Creating a necklace or bracelet. Each person can bring a bead for the mother-to-be. Women go around in a circle and read their blessing or

"A Blessing for Margo"

My mother wrote this blessing and read it to me during my birth blessing ceremony before my first child was born. *L'dor v'dor* means "from generation to generation" in Hebrew. This phrase honors and incorporates our Jewish heritage. I still cry every time I read this.

From generation to generation, l'dor v'dor
A new generation begins
with the birth of your baby.
Blessings for you, my daughter:
May you have a short, easy labor
milk that flows like honey
a baby who sleeps through the night.
May you learn to balance
sthira and *sukha*, firmness and gentleness,
through toilet training and temper tantrums.
May you keep your sense of humor
through homework hassles and
    language lessons.
May you practice patience and acceptance
when facing friendly fire and teen troubles.
May you give your child roots:
values and traditions of our family
and create new customs reflecting
    your marriage.
May your child grow up to be your friend
and bring you as much joy as you've given me,
for you are a blessing
and your baby will be a blessing too.
From generation to generation, l'dor v'dor
A new generation begins
with the birth of your baby.

say some positive words while stringing their bead. At the end, the pregnant woman can wear her necklace or bracelet infused with blessings from her friends.

Henna on the belly. Henna, a dye made from a flowering plant, is used to make beautiful designs on hands, feet, and sometimes bellies for rituals. It is nontoxic and lasts on your skin for one to two weeks. Drawing henna designs is a fun, artistic activity. Guests can help create a gorgeous image on the woman's pregnant belly.

Pampering the mama. Women can gather around the mother-to-be and soak her feet in aromatic water, massage her, and brush her hair.

When I organized a birth blessing ceremony for my dear friend Maria, I asked each woman to bring a flower (although some brought big bouquets) and a handwritten blessing for her. A large group of women gathered at Maria's home on a hot Sunday afternoon in July, and we all shared a delicious, healthy meal together. Afterward Maria sat on the sofa and we all encircled her. One by one, we went up and placed the flowers on or around her and read our blessings. Then we chanted to honor the fullness of life together. By the end, she was glowing from this shower of sweet blessings, love, and flowers.

ASANA PRACTICE

Balance Poses

Balance poses help you to find your center of gravity, which shifts in pregnancy. Balance poses show you where to put your attention and help draw your awareness back to your body and breath when your mind wanders. Increased focus, concentration, and centeredness, natural results of balance poses, are immensely helpful in labor.

Balance poses also improve coordination, increase strength, and help you develop stability. With regular practice, you may find yourself moving with grace and a sense of fluidity through all activities in your day, and also avoiding accidents and injuries.

The basis for these balance poses is a posture called Samasthiti or "Equal Standing Pose." However basic this pose may seem, it is wonderful for reestablishing proper alignment, building strength in the legs, and feeling stable. Always begin in Samasthiti and return to Samasthiti in between each pose. End these asanas with the basic squat as a counterpose. Be near a wall or use the support of a chair in case you lose your balance.

1. SAMASTHITI (EQUAL STANDING POSE)

- Stand with your feet a comfortable distance apart. Feel your feet planted firmly on the ground, your weight balanced on both feet.
- Relax your arms by your sides. Relax your shoulders back and down and keep your chest broad, open, and lifted.
- Take a deep breath. Imagine a string going from the top of your head to the sky, aligning your shoulders, hips, and ankles.
- Keep your chin parallel to the floor and your gaze forward.

2. TADASANA (MOUNTAIN POSE)

See page 109.

3. VRIKSHASANA (TREE POSE)

- Stand in Samasthiti, facing a wall or chair.
- Shift your weight to your left leg. Gently lift your right leg off the floor.
- Place the sole of your right foot on the inside of your left leg. It can be anywhere along the leg except on your knee. You can also place your foot flat on a chair.
- Fix your gaze on a point on the wall in front of you, at eye level.

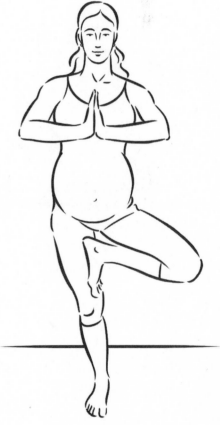

figure 20 **Vrikshasana** (Tree Pose)

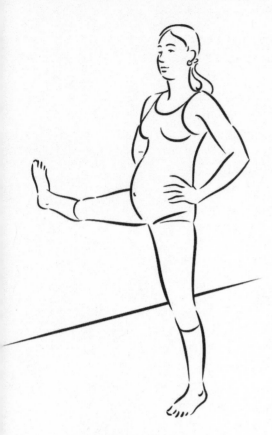

- Lift your hands up toward the sky, arms next to your ears. Then lower your hands and bring them together in prayer position in front of your heart.
- Hold this position for four long and smooth breaths. Release your foot to the floor and your arms by your side.
- Repeat on the other side.

4. UTTHITA HASTA PADANGUSHTHASANA (EXTENDED SIDE HAND TO BIG TOE POSE)

This is a pregnancy variation for the traditional pose.

- Start in Vrikshasana (Tree Pose), facing a wall or chair with your arms on your hips.
- If the sole of your foot is against your leg, place your hand under the bent-leg knee and move your leg so your heel is on a chair or your foot is flat against the wall.
- Place your hands on your hips and slightly lift your waist and chest to lift your heart center and create length in your torso.
- Lift from the center of your chest and feel your shoulder blades tucking toward each other. Stay for two breaths, feeling your center, your balance. Then release your foot to the floor.
- Repeat on the other side.

figure 21 **Utthita Hasta Padangushthasana** (Extended Side Hand to Big Toe Pose)

5. SQUATTING POSE

See page 122. *Skip this pose if you are thirty-four weeks or more along and your baby is in a breech position.*

6. NATARAJASANA (DANCING SIVA POSE)

- Begin in Samasthiti near a wall.
- Shift your weight onto your left leg.
- Bend your right knee, lifting your right foot toward your buttocks.
- Reach back with your right hand to grasp your foot in your palm.
- As you inhale, raise your left arm in front of you. You can place your hand on the wall for extra support.

- Balance and hold for three to five breaths. Focus your eyes on something to help keep you stable. Then lower your arm and release your leg to return to Samasthiti.
- Repeat on the other side.

7. SQUATTING POSE

See page 122. *Skip this pose if you are thirty-four weeks or more along and your baby is in a breech position.*

8. CAKRAVAKASANA (RUDDY GOOSE POSE)

See page 112.

9. SHAVASANA (CORPSE POSE)

See page 115. ⬥

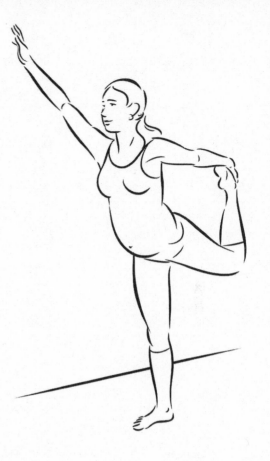

figure 22 **Natarajasana** (Dancing Siva Pose)

BREATHING PRACTICE

Silent Recitation Pranayama, So Hum

Traditionally, the silent recitation of sounds is used as a breathing exercise. It is a simple and subtle way to work with your breath.

In this practice you will use the same mantra you worked with in the third month as a meditation. You can see that there are many uses to these sacred phrases. *So hum* translates to "I am that," meaning "I am the light that dwells within me." This mantra helps to connect with the higher, unchanging, divine aspect of yourself.

Let your breath be long and smooth. If the practice becomes too strong, and you are finding it hard to catch your breath, back off and work below your breath's capacity.

- Begin by sitting in a comfortable position with your back straight. You can sit cross-legged on the floor, on a cushion in Sukhasana, or in a chair.
- Take a natural breath in and as you exhale, silently recite, "So." Just the sound "So." Do this two times.
- Take a natural breath in and as you exhale, silently recite, "So hum." Repeat two times. Remember this is silent recitation.

- Take a natural breath in and as you exhale, silently recite, "So hum so." Repeat two times. Let the length of your exhale match the length of your silent recitation.
- Take a natural breath in and as you exhale, silently recite, "So hum so hum." Do this twice.
- Inhale through your nose with your mouth closed. As you exhale, silently recite, "So hum so hum so." Repeat two times.
- Now inhale naturally and as you exhale, silently recite, "So hum so hum." Repeat two times.
- Inhale naturally and as you exhale, silently recite, "So hum so." Repeat two times.
- Inhale naturally and as you exhale, silently recite, "So hum." Do this two times.
- Finally, inhale naturally and as you exhale, silently recite, "So"—just where you began. Do this two times.

MEDITATION PRACTICE

Balance

In the busyness and intensity of life's demands, it's easy to lose your center. Balance in the body, breath, and mind help to cultivate equilibrium in all aspects of your life. This meditation practice helps to create steadiness in the mind and cultivate inner feelings of balance.

- Sit comfortably. Use blankets and pillows under your hips and buttocks to make yourself at ease. If you are feeling especially tired and would prefer to do this meditation lying down, you can lie on your side supported by pillows under your head and between your legs.
- Take a few deep breaths to settle in.
- Close your eyes and draw your attention inward. Bring your awareness to your breath. Take a few moments to observe the flow of your inhale and exhale.
- Ask yourself, "Do I feel connected to my center or scattered from my experiences today?" Whatever you experience is completely fine. Just notice.
- Ask yourself, "Can I find a place of stillness in myself?" Maybe that place is in the center of your body, such as your navel or your heart.

- Feel your breath moving in your body. Let your experiences be in the background of your mind. If your mind wanders, let it. Even though there may be a swirl of activity around you, root yourself in this place of stillness in your body.
- Focus your mind on that place of stillness and steadiness within yourself. Everything you are experiencing is floating on the stillness inside you.
- Now feel yourself moving into a state of balance. Balance, steadiness, calmness, and joy are always within you. You just need to tap into them.
- Bring your awareness back to your breath, noticing it moving in and out of your nose. Begin to notice the sounds around you. Slowly open your eyes and take a few minutes to adjust to your surroundings before getting up. 🌢

SOUND PRACTICE

Ayur Mantra

A mantra for health and nourishment, this chant is from the Yajur Veda. It is a blessing asking the divine forces to bestow upon us a long life that is filled with good health, clarity, and stability. This practice uses a few specific lines from the full chant.

- Sit in a comfortable position. You can sit cross-legged on the floor, on a cushion in Sukhasana, or in a chair.
- Let your breath lengthen your spine.
- For each of the following phrases, take a natural breath in, then exhale, reciting one line per exhale:

> Om ayur dhehi (om aayur day-hee)
> Om atmanam dhehi (om aatman-um day-hee)
> Om pratistham dhehi (om pratish-tam day-hee)

- Repeat each line, two more times.
- When finished, sit quietly for a few moments before getting up. 🌢

16

Month Nine

COMPLETION

You gain strength, courage, and confidence by every experience by which you really stop to look fear in the face. You are able to say to yourself, "I can take the next thing that comes along."
ELEANOR ROOSEVELT

Other women may have shared their birth stories with you. Some are magical beyond belief and others can be quite scary. Your midwife or doctor has tried to prepare you as much as she or he can. You may wonder if there is any way to truly prepare for giving birth. Can you be ready for the unexpected? It's like taking a trip: You pack your bags and bring what you think you may need, but if your trip takes an unexpected turn, you may need something new or different. You may need to shift, accommodate, and go with the flow. Birth is the same way. Staying flexible, open-minded, and empowered are essential preparations for what may come your way. Also, keep doing your practices, whatever they are: yoga, singing, meditation, breathing, and dancing. Continue doing whatever keeps you happy, relaxed, nourished, present in your body, and tapped into your inner strength.

Preparing for the birthing journey begins about six weeks before your expected due date. Daily activities and sleeping can become more difficult at this stage. Some women feel sensuous and juicy while others feel enormous and awkward. You are probably tired of your maternity clothes, but make it a point every day to wear fresh, clean, comfortable clothes. You will feel better.

If this is your first pregnancy, you may wish to make an extra effort to spend time around other new mothers and babies. Doing so can provide support and insight for what is to come. To become a little more "baby savvy," you can offer to help a friend or relative with her baby. Now is also the time to meet more frequently with your doula or whoever will be supporting you during labor.

There is a dual focus in late pregnancy: creating rest and relaxation coupled with staying strong and active. Integrate both aspects of self-care into your day. During this time of physical and emotional change and preparing for the birth and postpartum time, it is crucial to slow down your daily activities. It is very common to feel easily fatigued. Try to spend some time every day in restful silence and tranquility, such as in guided relaxation, meditation, watching a sunset, or taking a bath. Quiet time will calm the nervous system and allow your body and mind to unwind. Naps or early bedtimes promote rest, relaxation, and rejuvenation during this time—especially for Vata women. Kapha types often do better without naps and instead benefit from restorative yoga or gentle exercise to increase energy in the afternoon.

At the same time, keep up your strength and endurance, which you will rely on in labor. Labor is called "labor" because it is hard work! Countless women have said it is one of the most intense experiences of their lives and has taken every ounce of their energy. In my own labors, I was pushed to my limits, physically and emotionally, like never before. They were some of the most empowering experiences of my life, and like nothing else, they gave me more strength to face challenges.

Women in traditional cultures often work right up until the moment labor begins, and then squat under a tree and push out their child easily. Let visions of these women inspire you as you continue hiking up hills, swimming extra laps, or washing your windows. Of course, follow your healthcare provider's recommendations in late pregnancy, especially if you have high blood pressure or other health issues.

It is best to avoid pursuits that disperse your vital energy and have the potential to bring on labor prematurely, such as traveling or engaging in too many strenuous activities. Avoid holding back urine, gas, or bowel movements. Try not to get chilled or jarred, which disrupts the proper movement of *apana vayu*, the principle subdosha of Vata that rules childbirth.

It is completely normal and natural to feel a range of emotions that can change from day to day. You may feel immense excitement about meeting your new little one, while at the same time you may feel anxiety and uncertainty about your ability to give birth and what your new life will be like. In the last month of pregnancy, you can spend some time every day envisioning the birth you would like to have. Visualize your baby dropping into the birth canal headfirst and coming easily into the world.

Remember that your body has all the knowledge and strength it needs to birth your baby. Your baby will come into this world in whatever way it needs to. Always remember the bottom line: healthy mama, healthy baby.

Simple Practices: Abhyanga and Yoni Pichu

Two simple practices to help prepare for birth are the daily oil massage (abhyanga) and *yoni pichu.* Classical Ayurvedic texts advise that from the beginning of the ninth month of pregnancy until she gives birth, a woman should never remain without fat—meaning that she should anoint the body with oil and consume adequate healthy fats daily. If you have not continued with abhyanga, please revisit this nourishing and supportive endeavor. Massaging the belly, breasts, and perineum is key.

A practice called yoni pichu can be done daily in the last two to three weeks of pregnancy. Soak a tampon in oil (sesame and coconut are my favorites) or medicated ghee (such as licorice ghee, available from the Ayurvedic Institute; see resources section) and insert it daily into the yoni to lubricate the birth canal. Alternatively, you can apply and massage licorice ghee around the perineal area, the whole area from the vaginal opening to below the anus, to assist with delivery by lubricating and softening the cervix (or birth canal). Leave the oils on as long as they will stay on. You may want to wear a panty liner to prevent oil stains on your underwear.

Preparing for Birth and Postpartum

Many of the classical Ayurvedic texts talk about special huts or rooms for birth. In the modern versions of these places for giving birth—hospital rooms, birthing centers, or a place in your own home—you can take steps to create an environment that is tranquil, comforting, and reminds you of your connection to the earth and other women. You may want to have an inspiring picture or photograph, a sculpture, flowers, seashells, or prayer flags nearby. Choose objects that help you feel strong and clear.

I enjoyed having seashells with me to root me to the ocean waters, where

I take refuge and find renewal. I also had an aromatherapy mist handy (see chapter 17, page 182), a sprig of fresh rosemary from the garden, and I wore my favorite, most comfortable late-pregnancy dress.

Some women want to listen to soothing music or favorite songs to help them relax into their bodies. If you are at a hospital and wish to drown out other noises, you may want something that plays white noise or nature sounds like ocean waves. Make playlists ahead of time and bring your favorite device for listening to music.

Coconut water and electrolyte sports beverages are excellent to have on hand for refreshing and energizing drinks. Chyavanprash (an Ayurvedic rejuvenating herbal jam) can be eaten by the spoonful during early labor for a boost. Some women want to eat during early labor and others do not. It is best to have simple, easy-to-digest foods, such as a thermos of miso broth or other light soups, yogurt, dates, crackers, or fresh bread with ghee, on hand. Bring your favorite light snacks.

Preparing for the new baby by gathering all the necessities can be fun and exciting. Newborn babies need very few things, especially if you are planning on breastfeeding. It is a good idea to have newborn diapers, baby wipes, simple cotton newborn outfits, a few tiny hats, washcloths, and blankets. Make sure to wash all newborn items in a gentle, natural soap before they are next to your baby's delicate skin. You will need to have an infant car seat, which is good to install about a month before you are due. A sling or some sort of a baby carrier is fantastic to have from the beginning to keep your little one close to your body and free up your arms.

In chapter 17, you'll find additional preparation suggestions and an exercise to get you thinking about what else to include in your "tool bag" to support you during labor and birth.

This is also a good time to line up support for after the birth. Have a close friend arrange for others to cook for you, help with older children, and run errands. You may underestimate your needs now, but you will appreciate anything that lessens your load postpartum. Resting and bonding with your new baby should be your primary activities.

Eating and Digesting in the Last Month of Pregnancy

Paying attention to your digestion and diet can help you feel more comfortable at the end of pregnancy. It is quite common to experience digestive troubles in late pregnancy when the space for the intestines and other internal organs has shrunk from the size of the baby. Heartburn is a frequent complaint, along with constipation, gas, and indigestion. Eating smaller meals more often can help. Avoid heartburn-inducing foods (mainly Pitta-aggravating fare), such as tomatoes or chilies, and fried, fermented, and heavily spiced foods. It is a good idea to remain upright at least two hours after eating and to take a gentle stroll around the block. See appendix 1, "Remedies for Common Pregnancy Ailments," for more information.

Classical Ayurvedic texts recommend eating fresh foods that are creamy, soft, warm, and sweet in the last month. Eating foods that contain healthy fats is encouraged to nourish and lubricate the deeper tissues of the body. A warm rice cereal cooked with milk, cardamom, and ghee is a good example of all these qualities. It can prevent constipation and fluid retention while giving strength and promoting lubrication and elasticity in the body, all of which can help to facilitate an easy delivery.

Cardamom Rice Cereal

Ingredients
½ cup basmati rice
1 cup milk (or substitutes)
½ cup water
1 teaspoon cardamom powder
1 to 2 teaspoons ghee

Directions
In a strainer, rinse the rice under running water three times. Place rice, milk, and water in a small saucepan and bring to a boil. Lower the heat to medium-low, cover, and simmer until the rice is soft and has absorbed most of the liquid, about 20–25 minutes. Stir in the cardamom powder and let the rice sit, covered, for 5 minutes. Transfer the cereal to a bowl and stir in the ghee.

You can top with almond slivers, and drizzle honey or maple syrup on top. This makes a wonderful breakfast.

JOURNALING EXERCISE

Building Confidence

I can't help but think of Maria in *The Sound of Music*, belting out her song about confidence when she is leaving her known world at the abbey and entering a new situation caring for seven children. She sings about longing for adventure, feeling scared, trusting her heart, and ultimately, having confidence in herself.

Use this month to think honestly about your confidence in your ability to give birth. Take out your journal and ask yourself:

- How am I feeling about my ability to birth my baby?
- If I'm not feeling confident, what would help me feel confident?

Recognize your insecurities and take steps to move in the opposite direction. Talk with your partner, friend, doula, labor support, doctor, or midwife about your fears, support, and what you need. Acknowledge your strengths.

Keep doing your yoga practices every day. Let the strength in your body, especially your posture, build your confidence. ◖

ASANA PRACTICE
Integration

This movement practice combines many of the poses from previous chapters into one sequence. If this practice is done quickly, it can be invigorating and stimulating, making it ideal for morning time. If it is done at a slower, more relaxed pace, it is best before dinner or bedtime. Try both and notice how you feel. Also, feel free to return to any of the previous asana practices. Strive for a practice every day.

1. Tadasana (Mountain Pose) page 109
2. Virabhadrasana (Warrior Pose) page 110
3. Squatting Pose page 122
4. Trikonasana (Triangle Pose) page 145
5. Cakravakasana (Ruddy Goose Pose) page 112
6. Adho Mukha Shvanasana (Downward Facing Dog Pose) page 113
7. Balasana (Child's Pose) page 131
8. Supta Baddha Konasana (Reclining Bound Angle Pose) page 133
9. Shavasana (Corpse Pose) page 115 ◖

BREATHING PRACTICE
Relaxing and Calming the Breath

The relaxing and calming breath recommended for the first month of pregnancy is also excellent in late pregnancy, as it can help decrease the anxiety that can creep up as you get closer to your due date. Follow the instructions from the breathing practice in month one (page 83). Make sure you are completely comfortable before beginning the exercise. You may need extra pillows or blankets at this stage of pregnancy. Also, feel free to return to any of the other breathing practices in this book. ◖

MEDITATION PRACTICE

Flower Blooming Meditation

This meditation can help you visualize a birth that happens as smoothly and gently as the opening of a flower.

If you have a clear image in your mind of a particular bright, beautiful flower in full bloom, please use that for this meditation. You may wish to find a picture from a magazine, a photo album, or the Internet, or use an actual flower to inspire your vision. Place the image in front of you before you begin.

- Sit comfortably with your back upright, either on a cushion or in a chair. Or if you are feeling especially tired, find a restful reclining position supported with pillows or blankets, but make sure to keep the mind alert so you don't fall asleep.
- Look at the image of your flower and then gently close your eyes. Turn your attention inward.
- Take several slow, deep breaths to bring your awareness to your life force—your breath, prana.
- Feel your breath move in and out of your nostrils.
- Feel your breath going to your belly and to your baby. Bring your awareness to an image of your baby: he or she is head down in your body—and smiling.
- Envision your baby dropping lower into your pelvis, getting ready to come into the world.
- Picture yourself feeling strong and confident, yet relaxed and receptive for what may come.
- Let each breath open up your body.
- Picture your bright, beautiful flower in your mind. You are the bright, beautiful flower. As you breathe, you bloom, opening completely, and your baby moves lower and lower, smoothly making his or her way out of your body.
- If your mind wanders, allow each breath to connect you back to your visualization—feeling relaxed and strong, blooming, opening, meeting your baby, holding your baby in your arms.
- Allow yourself to go deeper and create other positive visions for yourself in labor.

• Bring your awareness back to the breath moving in and out of your nose. Begin to notice the sounds around you. Slowly open your eyes and take a few minutes to adjust to your surroundings before getting up. 🌢

SOUND PRACTICE

Purnamadah, "Honoring the Wholeness of Life"

This is a prayer for self-knowledge and a prayer that honors the fullness of life and the spirit of wholeness in all things. I love this chant for late pregnancy, when the belly is so round and full of life, because it helps women connect to the source of life and all things.

I guided many women in this chant at my dear friend's blessing ceremony. It was a joyful time as we blessed our friend, full of baby and surrounded by everyone who loved her, on her way into motherhood. She seemed so filled with love afterward.

The direct translation of the chant is:

That is whole; this is whole.
From the whole, this whole came.
Remove this whole from that whole,
What remains is still whole.

• Sit in a comfortable position. You can sit cross-legged on the floor, on a cushion in Sukhasana, or in a chair.
• Let the breath lengthen the spine.
• For each of the following phrases, take a natural breath in, then exhale, reciting one line per exhale:

Purnamadah (poor-nah-mah-dah)
Purnamidam (poor-nah-mee-dum)
Purnat (poor-naat)
Purnamudachyate (poor-nah-moo-datch-yuh-tay)
Purnasya (poor-nas-yah)
Purnamadaya (poor-nah-mah-daa-yah)
Purnameva (poor-nah-may-vaa)

Vashishyate (va-shish-yah-tay)
Purnamadah purnamidam
Purnat purnamudachyate
Purnasya purnamadaya
Purnameva vashishyate

- Repeat the whole chant, if time permits.
- When finished, sit quietly for a few moments before getting up.

PART THREE

Birth and Postpartum

17

The Journey of Birth

<blockquote>
Birthing is the most profound initiation to spirituality a woman can have.
ROBIN LIM
</blockquote>

Early Labor

"The time is finally here!" I excitedly thought as early labor began with my second child. Like his older sister, my son had stayed in my womb past his due date, and each passing day had seemed like an eternity, filled with great anticipation. Now I felt some contractions, but they were quite weak. My husband and I turned on a movie for a little distraction and the contractions completely stopped. We couldn't believe it. We turned off the movie and took a walk, which brought the labor back. Watching the sun drop lower on the horizon, we stopped every few minutes for me to breathe deeply and squeeze the life out of my husband's hand. We walked home; I performed a short oil massage, showered, and got dressed. Before we knew it, we were gathering our belongings and calling our doula and doctor and heading to the hospital.

Early labor is when there are mild contractions lasting from thirty to ninety seconds. These contractions can feel like pressure in the pelvis, menstrual cramping, or a dull backache. Women can often carry on a conversation, eat a light meal, wash a few dishes, and rest during this phase, which can last from a few hours to several days. Walking is very useful in early labor to help the baby move down and to help labor progress. With time, the contractions get stronger, closer together, more regular, and longer lasting.

I assisted my dear friend Susanna at her birth. I went to her home as soon as she called me to let me know she was in early labor. When I arrived, I inhaled the aroma of a fresh pot of miso soup as I helped her off the sofa and into the bathtub. She spent her entire early labor in warm waters and the comfort of her own home, which helped her to deeply relax and allowed her to dilate. Every so often, she added more warm water to the tub, splashed it over her belly, and consciously breathed through each contraction. In her own words, "The warm bathing waters eased each contraction, and I remember just looking down at my large belly awaiting the miracle to arrive. I was fortunate to not labor so long. Long, deep breaths, just riding the tidal waves of my own biorhythm. And of course your hand was there to comfort me during the most magical moment a woman can pass through on her journey to embody her deep feminine, the birth of a child."

Ayurvedic texts tell us that when a woman enters early labor, it is best to anoint her with oil, bathe her in warm water, and dress her in clean, comfortable clothes. A loose-fitting dress is preferable because it makes it easier for the woman to move and for her caregivers to check her dilation.

Yoga for Labor

Yoga is an incredible boon to a woman in early and active labor. Consciously breathing and moving your body can help you feel more comfortable, focus your mind, and help the baby shift positions and move lower into your pelvis. Moving around can also increase your sense of control and may decrease or prevent the need for analgesia (drugs for pain relief). A few beneficial yogic practices are:

Breath awareness. Tune into your breath and deepen the inhalation and exhalation to calm your system. Revisit the "Relaxing and Calming the Breath" practice from chapter 6 (page 83). Perform this practice sitting cross-legged on your bottom or lying on your side with pillows between your knees and under your head for support.

Cakravakasana. Slowly move in and out of this pose (see page 112) to encourage the baby to move and shift its position if necessary. It also just feels wonderful.

Upavishta Konasana and Baddha Konasana. Practice these postures (pages 132 and 123), with the support of a bolster or blankets, to help open the pelvis.

These three asanas also facilitate maximum comfort and effectiveness in labor and allow access to a woman's back for massage to relieve pain.

Chanting or singing your favorite mantra or song can also help you focus your mind and connect with your strength.

EXERCISE

Reviewing Yoga to Help You in Labor with Your Partner/Labor Support

Go back through part 2 and review yoga postures with your partner and/ or the person who will be supporting you in labor. Review the three poses mentioned in the previous section and any others that brought relief from discomfort, helped you to connect with your breath, or just felt good. Go over how to move in the postures and make any adaptations for comfort. For example, you may need more blankets to sit on or for support at this stage of pregnancy. Make sure your support people know these asanas well, so they can help you do them when you are in labor and remind you which ones you like. Review songs, chants, and meditations that were helpful to you as well, so your support people can guide and remind you. ◗

Support During Active Labor

In the second stage of labor, called *active labor*, contractions strengthen and accelerate, helping the cervix to dilate. During active labor, your partner or labor support can do all they can to keep your spirits up. Drinking water, having water misted on you, and bathing in warm water can promote relaxation and relieve pain and anxiety during labor. During the intensity of labor with my second child, I retreated to a birthing tub, which felt heavenly. The warm water helped me to deeply relax, so I stayed in the tub until just before it was time to begin pushing.

Warmed oil, such as sesame, can be lightly massaged over your waist, pelvis, hips, and legs to alleviate pain and help your baby move down. Wherever there is pain, Vata dosha is involved. This is especially true in childbirth, since the baby's exit is governed by apana vayu. Warm oil massage is invaluable to soothe Vata, as well as increase your comfort in labor.

Encouraging words can help you feel happy and empowered, help your heart to open, and help your body, especially your cervix, relax. I love this short story, taken from *Ina May's Guide to Childbirth*, because it illuminates the power of the mind-body connection:

> She had been sitting on her bed in the first stage of labor (during which the cervix is opening), encircled in her husband's arms. He whispered in her ear, "You're marvelous!" and she was sure she felt her cervix open when she heard his words.
>
> "Please say that again!" she told him.
>
> He repeated the words, and she again felt her cervix open.
>
> "I *know* you're going to think I'm crazy," she said, addressing both him and her midwife, "but would you keep saying that?"
>
> Her husband, joined by her midwife, kept up the chant. Soon, her cervix was completely dilated, and she pushed her baby out.

During the intensity of labor, don't wish it to be over! Try to stay in the present moment. Let yourself be loud, earthy, primal, and raw. Surrender to the magic of birthing. Tell your baby it is safe to come into the world. Dance, move your body, and *breathe*. Always come back to your breath. Breathe through every contraction. Whether you took a special class to learn breathing techniques for labor or practiced yoga throughout your pregnancy, your breath will guide you and be your anchor while you ride the waves of each contraction. *Every contraction brings you closer to your baby.*

The pushing stage of labor can last from fifteen minutes to several hours. Licorice ghee can be used for perineal massage, and warm compresses can also be used to soften the perineal tissues, reduce inflammation, prevent tearing, and decrease the need for an episiotomy. Some women enjoy massage and compresses, and others don't like being touched. Neither option has been confirmed effective or ineffective; using massage, compresses, or using nothing is solely maternal preference.

You may enjoy squatting, being on your hands and knees, lying on your side, or even sitting on a toilet to push your baby out.

Marma Points to Assist with Labor

Marma points are pressure points throughout the body where prana—life force or energy—is concentrated. *Marma* translates to "vulnerable" or "sensitive" area. Similar to acupuncture points, they are part of Ayurvedic science. When marmas are stimulated, they can enhance health and provide information for the diagnosis and treatment of disease. Marmas are located and measured in "finger units," or *angulas*.

Working with the subtle currents of prana that run through the marmas can ease the pain of labor and assist with the whole birthing process. The chart "Marma Points to Assist with Labor" highlights some marma points that can be employed during labor. *It is very important that these points are not stimulated during pregnancy (unless under the guidance of a skilled practitioner), but used only when labor is imminent or has begun, because they can encourage labor.* Massage a point in a circular motion with firm pressure for about five minutes.

Marma Points to Assist with Labor

NAME OF MARMA	LOCATION IN THE BODY	USE IN LABOR	ADDITIONAL INFORMATION
URDHVA SKANDHA	On the upper shoulders at the superior aspect of the trapezius muscle.	Sends messages to the uterus to contract. Can be used in early labor or in a labor that is not progressing.	Also useful for relieving stress and calming the mind. Pressure on this marma stimulates the downward flow of energy, apana vayu.
GULPHA MARMA	Consists of two points located on the lateral and medial parts of the ankle bone. Lateral gulpha is in a depression below the lateral malleolus. Medial gulpha is one angula inferior and one angula posterior to the tip of the medial malleolus.	Relieves tension, stress, and lower back pain. Can be used in early and active labor. Pacifies Kapha-type emotions, such as holding and stagnancy.	
JANU MARMA	Consists of two points located on the posterior and anterior aspects of the knee joint. Posterior janu is at the midpoint of the popliteal crease. Anterior janu is at the center of the patella.	Releases spasms of the uterus and helps with pelvic pain.	Stimulating this marma can relieve dizziness.

Marma Points to Assist with Labor, continued

NAME OF MARMA	LOCATION IN THE BODY	USE IN LABOR	ADDITIONAL INFORMATION
TRIKA MARMA	Located at the tip of the coccyx.	Useful for labor pain.	Useful for treating many reproductive system disorders. This marma is associated with the seat of dormant kundalini and is intimately related to root chakra.
NABHI MARMA	A large marma region located at and around the center of the belly button. There are also four additional marmas surrounding the navel.	Can facilitate labor in general.	Through the nabhi marma the baby receives oxygen and nutrients from the mother. Sometimes just placing the hands in this area is enough to gently stimulate this marma.

EXERCISE

Finding the Marmas on Your Body
with Your Partner/Labor Support

Refer to the "Marma Points to Assist with Labor" table and find these marma points on your own body. Have your partner and/or labor support become familiar with where these points are. Simply place your finger on the point but remember *not* to apply pressure before labor. To get a feel for them, you can practice massaging the points on someone who is not pregnant. Review them a few times. ◗

Aromatherapy During Labor

Aromatherapy is an extraordinary tool for transforming a labor environment and supporting a woman's birthing journey. Essential oils—powerful, highly concentrated extracts of plants made from flowers, leaves, seeds, roots, trees, and resins—have been used for thousands of years by cultures around the world for attaining health, longevity, and spiritual insight.

The sense of smell activates the limbic system, the most primitive aspect of the brain that bypasses logical reasoning and thinking. The limbic system is directly connected to parts of the brain that control heart rate, blood pressure, stress levels, breathing, memory, and hormone balance. This relationship helps explain why smells often trigger emotions, and how using essential oils can have profound physiological and psychological effects.

Let your nose guide you. Smell different oils and make a birth blend or purchase several oils to have available, and smell them once you're in labor to decide which ones to use at the time. Essential oils can be mixed into massage oil, added to a warm bath, distributed through a spray bottle or diffuser, or put on a washcloth to inhale. For more information, refer to appendix 6, "How to Use Essential Oils Safely and Effectively."

The chart "Essential Oils for Labor" lists oils that have been used empirically for specific birthing situations. This is not an exhaustive list, and you may have different experiences and choose to use different oils.

Essential Oils for Labor

TO HELP:	USE:
RELIEVE PAIN	lavender, clary sage, frankincense, wintergreen, peppermint, balsam fir
STRENGTHEN CONTRACTIONS	clary sage, jasmine
A STALLED LABOR	clary sage, myrrh
RELIEVE EXHAUSTION, REFRESH AND UPLIFT	citrus oils like sweet orange, lemon, and grapefruit; peppermint and evergreens oils like fir and spruce
CALM AND RELAX	lavender, neroli, rose, frankincense, sandalwood, and geranium
REMEMBER YOUR STRENGTH AND CONNECT TO OTHER WOMEN WHO HAVE GIVEN BIRTH BEFORE YOU	rosemary

EXERCISE

What Else Is in Your Tool Bag?

Giving birth is an intimate and personal experience. You will have your own special things you would like to have with you. This is your time to think about it and gather your necessities, both inspirational and practical. Smell different essential oils and make your blends. Burn a CD or make a playlist. Review chapter 16 for other ideas I mentioned. Place everything together in a bag. Communicate your wishes with your partner and/or labor support so they know what you would like in your tool bag, as well as other ways they can support you during labor. ⬧

There are no right or wrong ways to give birth. Every woman has the right to choose to give birth naturally. Natural childbirth allows

Aromatherapy Birth Mist

Here is a recipe for a mixture of pure water and essential oils that you can mist on and around you while in labor. I recently used this mist at my friend's birth. We (my friend, her doula, and I) loved misting the room whenever the energy got stale. It completely refreshed, uplifted, and transformed the atmosphere.

Ingredients

1 (4-ounce) bottle, glass or plastic, with a mister top
Just less than 4 ounces of purified water
18 drops lavender essential oil
12 drops geranium essential oil
9 drops clary sage essential oil
3 drops chamomile essential oil
1 drop frankincense essential oil

Directions

Mix the water and oils in the mister bottle. Shake well, mist, and inhale deeply.

You can also add other oils or begin with smaller amounts of these oils and slowly increase the number of drops until you find a combination that is right for you.

a woman to actively participate in labor, helps her feel in control of her body, and be alert and feel all the sensations of her experience. This book highlights natural methods to facilitate unmedicated birth, including prebirth visualizations and marma-point massage, yoga, labor support, breath awareness, and aromatherapy during labor. With the right tools and support, women often feel empowered and deeply satisfied by natural childbirth.

In today's world, women have many resources available for difficult labors. Keeping this in mind will support and comfort you and increase your confidence in your ability to birth your baby, however it may happen.

Immediately After Birth

After the exhilaration and intensity of birth, it is best to keep you and your baby warm and comfortable. Place the baby directly on your chest (or your partner's chest if you are unable) right after she emerges. Rest together in quiet and darkness, for as long as possible. This is a crucial time of connection after the birthing journey. There is no need to rush into cleaning and testing the baby unless it is medically indicated.

According to Ayurvedic texts, the best time to cut the umbilical cord is once the pulsation ends. This helps with the transfer of ojas from the mother to the baby.

The mother can receive an oil massage and sponge bath, and she can put on fresh clothing and drink a mug of warm tea or milk. After a mild and gentle washing with water, warm coconut or sesame oil can be massaged into the baby's skin, especially on the fontanels. Then the baby can be wrapped in a warm blanket, with her head covered. Breastfeeding, the best food for the baby, is the natural next step.

The wisdom of Ayurveda, yoga, and the natural world can help you and your baby through this life-transforming stage. Just as they guided your pregnancy and birth, they can inspire radiant health through your post-partum time and well beyond.

18

Gentle Beginnings

THE FIRST TWO MONTHS POSTPARTUM

*The best and most beautiful things in the world cannot be seen nor touched
but are felt in the heart.*
HELEN KELLER

Staring into the tender eyes of your new baby for the first time is mysteriously wonderful. You have intimately housed this soul within your body for the past nine months, and she will continue to be closely connected to you for as long as you walk the earth. The mother-child bond is inseparable, extraordinary, and profound. With post-birthing fatigue and bliss, try to savor these precious fleeting moments as you move into your new lives together.

The initial postpartum time is a delicate juncture for you as a new mother and for your family. It is a time of healing and transition physically, emotionally, socially, and psychologically. After giving birth, a woman is as fragile, energetically open, and vulnerable as her newborn infant. You are recovering from labor and birth and adjusting to include a new member of your family. Your baby is adapting to her new environment—life outside the womb, her parents, and siblings. Love, patience, and gentleness are essential for everyone's health and harmony within your home.

In the first six weeks to many months after the birth, the optimum activities for the mother and baby are resting, bonding, healing, receiving nourishment, and allowing their growing relationship to flourish. You have been through a lot. Resting is vital to recovering from the intensity of birth and to adjusting to the demands of nursing and tending to your little one every couple of hours, around the clock.

Our modern society likes to rush. But when you take time to slow down, *especially* in the initial postpartum time, you bestow many benefits on yourself and your baby for short- and long-term health. Rushing back into household and work responsibilities can set you up for exhaustion, depletion, slower recovery time, and postpartum depression.

Many cultures around the world have postpartum rituals and diets for health, healing, and vitality. Traditional women in India, Mexico, Guatemala, and Japan, for example, pass down their postpartum traditions to their children. They alter their diets to consume warm, soupy foods with extra oil and traditional digestive spices. They take herbs to stabilize hormones and help with lactation and digestion. The mother and baby are massaged, and the mother is excused from her daily responsibilities and cared for completely. This time is not viewed as one of self-indulgence for the mother; these cultures know it is a vital time for both the mother's and the newborn's health and that taking care of them will eventually benefit all of society. The saying goes, "When Mama is happy, all are happy."

Just as every woman's experience of pregnancy is unique, so is every woman's postpartum time. Dr. Aviva Romm, a midwife, says, "Many consider six weeks to be an arbitrary and terribly limited definition of time allocated for the postpartum, recognizing that it takes much longer than six weeks to fully physically and emotionally recover from the demands placed on a woman by pregnancy and birth, and much longer than this to adjust to the demands of motherhood." I have seen some women moving through this time with great support, which allows for a quicker recovery and adjustment. Others can take several months to years (yes, years) to recover from pregnancy and birth and settle into the demands of motherhood.

The first three months after birth have been referred to by many as the "fourth trimester," since it can take another three months after the baby arrives for the mother to feel integrated, find rhythms for sleep and eating, and adjust to a new daily life. Some say that postpartum lasts for two years. Your adjustment period will last as long it needs to for your particular family. Accepting this uniqueness is a key piece of your recuperation.

Guidelines for Mom's and Baby's Health and Happiness

Following is a list of ideas to create health and happiness in the initial six weeks after birth, although these ideas can be used for as long as desired. By following these suggestions, your recovery and rejuvenation are greatly enhanced, and the chances of developing postpartum depression are considerably reduced.

- Sleep when your baby sleeps. Don't be tempted to try to get everything done while your baby naps. Use this time to rest and sleep before she wakes and needs you, or your other children need you.
- For the first three weeks, stay in bed as much as you can and as close to your baby as you can.
- Minimize cold drafts, wind, bright lights, noise, and media stimulation.
- Minimize visits and the length of time visitors stay.
- Try to stay inside with your baby for six weeks. Shield yourself and your baby's delicate nervous system from the outside world until he is a little older. If you go outside, cover your baby's head and ears.
- Don't lift anything heavier than your baby.
- Pay attention to your diet. (See "Postpartum Diet" later in this chapter.) Do not attempt to diet or skimp on your calories now. The food you ingest is deeply nourishing both you and your baby.
- Massage yourself or have someone else massage you daily with copious amounts of warm oil, and follow that with a hot bath, if possible. (See "An Essential Practice: The Ayurvedic Self-Massage" in chapter 4, page 68.) Plain sesame or almond oil or medicated ashwagandha/bala oil (see Banyan Botanicals in the resources section) is a good choice.
- Pay special attention to massaging your abdomen. Afterward, wrap a clean cloth around your belly, compressing it slightly to prevent a hollow space from forming where the baby was and to encourage organs and tissues to return to their proper places. You can use a lightweight cotton cloth or scarf about four to five yards long.
- Massage your baby. (See "Ayurvedic Baby Massage" in this chapter.)
- Line up as much help as you can for food shopping, cooking, cleaning, errands, and assisting with older children. Also arrange help so you can have time to bathe, shower, nap, or take quiet

Postpartum Herbal Sitz Bath

A postpartum herbal sitz bath is a brew of soothing and healing herbs for your perineum. Herbs that are uplifting, astringent, and antiseptic can reduce inflammation, and aid tissue repair and overall recovery. You can purchase a premade mix (see Motherlove products in the resources section) or prepare your own, using the following recipe.

Ingredients

1 ounce calendula flowers
1 ounce comfrey leaf
1 ounce yarrow flowers
1 ounce lavender flowers
½ ounce sage leaves
4 quarts water

Directions

Mix all the herbs together.

Bring 4 quarts of water to a boil in a large pot. Turn off heat and add 1 ounce of the herb mixture. Cover and steep for thirty minutes. Strain the herbs. Use immediately and/or refrigerate.

It will keep for two days.

To Use

Add 2 quarts of the liquid to a shallow (up to your hips) bath. Some women also enjoy adding ½ cup of sea salt to their bath for its astringent and antiseptic actions. Soak for 10 to 30 minutes. Repeat daily in the first week or two after birth.

You can also place this brew in a squirt bottle and spray on your perineum after going to the bathroom.

---

personal time. Allow yourself to be nurtured by others.

- Have someone you know well and trust be available for support, listening, and encouragement.
- Don't rush anything. It takes time to heal. Learn your baby's cues and find your rhythms together.
- Drink a tall glass of room temperature or warm water every time you breastfeed.
- Consult with your doctor or midwife before returning to any exercise programs. Gentle stretching and breathing are probably okay.
- Go to bed early, by 10:00 p.m.

In the first two weeks after both of my children were born, I did a short ritual for my self-renewal. It began with tenderly giving my newborn to my husband, friend, or mother to hold for a half hour to an hour, after nursing. I boiled a large pot of water to steep herbs for Postpartum Nourishing Tea (page 195) and a sitz bath. While the herbs were steeping, I massaged myself with warm medicated oil, which was deeply nourishing and grounding. Then I did a sitz bath, followed by a hot shower. The water rinsed away so much! Excess breast milk, sweat, and fatigue left me every time. I ended with wrapping a scarf around my belly and putting on fresh clothing. This short and precious time away from caring for my baby left me recharged to meet the demands of motherhood.

JOURNALING EXERCISE

Writing Your Birth Story

Birthing your child is a profound experience. Processing the details of your birth can be a vital piece of your postpartum recovery and can ease the transition from pregnancy into motherhood. Take a deep breath and write down your birth story. If you forget some of the details, ask someone who was with you. Recall:

- who was there with you
- how you felt in the different stages of labor
- how long you were in labor
- your most joyful memory
- whether you had any disappointments
- any insights that arose from the process

Take your time, do not limit the story's length, and don't hold back tears or laughter. Then read it to someone dear to you. ◊

Postpartum Diet

Typically, Ayurveda does not suggest a one-size-fits-all approach to anything, especially diet. However, there are particular time frames, including the postpartum time, that are ruled by certain doshas and warrant a general diet across the board. These overall Vata-reducing recommendations benefit all women during this time, and each woman can make her own special adjustments.

The postpartum time is governed by Vata dosha for several reasons. First, the act of giving birth is ruled by apana vayu, Vata's principle subdosha, which becomes weak from this monumental event. After the baby leaves the body, a large emptiness is left where the baby resided for nine months. This area can feel tender, and needs to be appropriately cared for by following a Vata-reducing diet and lifestyle. Second, after delivery of the baby, the mother's digestive system is usually weakened and delicate, which typically can bounce back from Vata palliation. Finally, Vata rules junctures, such as those of the day (sunrise, sunset), season, and stage of life. Postpartum is a transition from pregnancy into motherhood that, again, responds well to a Vata-reducing program.

Freshly prepared, warm, moist, nourishing, grounding, non-spicy, easy-to-digest foods are best, such as porridges, soups, and stews. Gentle spices, such as cinnamon, cardamom, fennel, saffron, basil, oregano, turmeric, cumin, coriander, and black pepper, kindle the digestive fire. Healthy fats are needed for milk production, hormonal balance, and energy. Use ghee and oils, such as olive, coconut, sesame, and flax, generously. Some classical texts suggest consuming meat (chicken, turkey, or fish) soups after about twelve days, based on a woman's strength and her digestive power. This can be nourishing if you are an omnivore.

Baked, steamed, and sautéed vegetables, such as carrots, spinach, asparagus, and zucchini, are good options. Veggies in the *Brassica* family (such as cabbage, cauliflower, broccoli, and kale) are best avoided initially, due to their gas-producing qualities. This can be challenging if they are staples in your diet. However, cooking these veggies in a Vata-reducing way (well-cooked, spiced, and oiled) can alleviate much of the discomfort due to gas.

Moistened whole grains, soaked nuts, and whole milk dairy products are also beneficial (see the complete Vata food guidelines in appendix 2). Try to avoid dry, crunchy snacks, such as crackers and chips; cold, raw, or frozen food and drinks; coffee, soda, chocolate, and alcohol.

The table "Foods to Favor and Avoid in Postpartum" summarizes key elements of the ideal postpartum diet, while the table "Sample Postpartum Meals" offers more ideas.

Foods to Favor and Avoid in Postpartum

FAVOR	warm, well-cooked, moist, unctuous foods
	mild spices such as cinnamon, ginger, and basil
	salty and sweet tastes
	sweet, fresh fruits and well-cooked vegetables
	grains such as oats, rice, and wheat
	lentils, mung beans, and aduki beans
	most dairy, especially warm
	most nuts
	ample amounts of sesame oil, olive oil, and ghee
AVOID	frozen, cold foods and beverages
	raw foods
	dried fruits and vegetables
	nightshades such as tomatoes and peppers
	dry, powdered milk

Sample Postpartum Meals

BREAKFAST	LUNCH/DINNER	SNACKS AND SWEETS
Cream of rice or wheat cereal, oatmeal, or other hot spiced grain cereal with ghee, milk, and raw sugar or honey	Red lentil dal and kitchari (pages 256 and 49)	Blanched and roasted almonds or walnuts
	Vegetable soups and stews	Pudding with milk or coconut milk
	Roasted carrots, beets, and winter squash	Cottage cheese (room temperature)
Stewed or baked fruits with spices such as cinnamon and cardamom	Asparagus, carrots, and zucchini sautéed in ghee	Avocado on warm whole grain bread or tortilla
	Aduki bean stew	
	Chicken soup with fresh ginger	Date and almond shakes
Warm, spiced milk	Basmati rice, quinoa, or barley	Fresh squeezed juices
	Warm pasta salads with basil and oregano	Yogurt shakes
Roasted nuts and seeds	Vegetable and herb quiche	Baked bananas with ginger, cardamom, and coconut

Rachel birthed her first child at forty-eight years old! She followed a strict Vata-reducing diet for her first two months postpartum and found that the suggested foods and preparations were exactly what she was craving. She noticed that the extra fats and emphasis on well-cooked, warming foods helped her to regain her strength and build up her resistance again. Rachel also found that the Vata-reducing lifestyle recommendations helped her to feel grounded and much less anxious. She was glowing and looking healthy again after two months, when I saw her last.

You will learn quite quickly which foods are working well for you and which are not by your response and especially by your baby's response. A small amount of gas can be normal. Symptoms of excessive gas from your baby are crying, spitting up, and certain movements such as pulling her knees into her chest or arching her back to relieve gas pains. Common culprits are foods in the *Brassica* family (especially if they are not well-cooked, oiled, and spiced), onions and garlic, hard cheeses, eggs, tofu, meat, beans, alcohol, spicy food, or too much fruit. It is important to try to remedy digestive upsets, and make your diet as nutritious as possible, since your baby's health depends on it.

Diet and Breast Milk

What the mother eats and drinks significantly affects the quality and quantity of her breast milk. Ayurveda places great emphasis on the mother's diet if she is breastfeeding. A woman's emotional state affects her breast

Remedies for Gas

Digestive Tea: Boil 2 cups of water. Add ½ teaspoon each of whole cumin, coriander, and fennel seeds. Let the seeds steep for 5 minutes. Remove from heat, strain, and drink warm or at room temperature.

Fennel Remedy: Dry-roast fennel seeds in a cast-iron skillet until they are slightly brown and you can smell their aroma. Chew a small pinch well after meals.

Ginger Remedy: Grate fresh ginger until you have 1 teaspoon of pulp. Add 1 teaspoon of lime juice and take immediately after eating.

milk as well. Anxiety, worry, or emotional turmoil can disturb the baby.

According to Ayurveda, a mother's ojas continues to be transferred to her baby through her breast milk, providing superior support to the baby's immune system. Therefore, it is very important for nursing mothers to consume healthy, nutritious food.

Years ago while in Peru, I stumbled upon a breastfeeding rally. Hundreds of indigenous women with long braids and colorful shawls carried their babies in slings and held signs saying ¡Viva La Leche Materna! ("Long Live Maternal Milk!"). I was surprised and wondered why they would need to fight to breastfeed their babies. Later I had a conversation with my mother, who told me that her generation of women was discouraged from breastfeeding and was sent home from the hospital with formula. Fifty years ago, another woman I know was given medication to dry up her breast milk because a nurse told her she would not be able to nurse. What a crime!

"No other milk can be compared with mother's milk for proper growth and development of the child," says the *Ayurvediya Prasuti-Tantra Evam Stri-Roga*, an Ayurvedic text for women's health. Breast milk is considered the perfect food for babies and it is what the human baby has evolutionarily adapted to expect. It has been scientifically proven that "Breast is Best!" Today, the American Academy of Pediatrics (AAP) has determined that breastfeeding is the ideal means to feed and nurture an infant. The AAP and the World Health Organization (WHO) recommend exclusive breastfeeding for about the first six months of a baby's life, followed by breastfeeding in combination with appropriate complementary foods until up to two years of age or beyond, as mutually desired by mother and baby. It's truly extraordinary to see an infant grow from its mother's milk.

Breastfeeding contributes to optimal health, growth, and development of the immune system, nervous system, skeletal system, and brain. It protects infants from a host of diseases and imbalances, and gives them a rock-solid foundation for the rest of their life. One of breastfeeding's greatest, yet immeasurable gifts is the tender love and intimacy shared between mother and babe. Nursing can become a meditation as you sit down, breathe deeply, and do nothing else except offer nourishment to your little one.

Breastfeeding can be challenging and painful at first, but don't give up. There are many resources available today to assist with breastfeeding. Nurses in hospitals are often trained to help get women started, and lactation consultants are available throughout the country to assist with techniques for a good latch-on. Women with inverted nipples can successfully breastfeed with a little extra effort to coax their nipples out and/or possibly by wearing a nipple shield (a small plastic nipple worn over a mother's nipple). Treating breastfeeding problems, such as insufficient quantity, infections, and cracked nipples, is beyond the scope of this book, but they can be remedied with herbs, diet, and lifestyle changes.

I had my own difficulties latching both my children on in the first weeks of life. It was very frustrating for both of us, but with persistence and support we overcame the initial struggle. I happily nursed both of my children until they were two years old.

Not all women can breastfeed. If you had a mastectomy, have an active infectious disease, or if you adopted a baby or had a surrogate, you can still nurture your baby by holding him in your arms, providing skin-to-skin contact, and giving him a bottle with loving hands. Feeding can still become a meditation. Sit quietly, breathe deeply, and stare into your baby's eyes, allowing him to become your object of meditation. Just think of how many opportunities you will have to meditate with your baby nursing every few hours.

Just as your diet sustained and nourished you and your baby in pregnancy, it continues to do so during breastfeeding. You still need more calories, but

Ayurvedic Postpartum Rejuvenating Elixir

The Ayurvedic herbs shatavari and ashwagandha are potent rejuvenators. Ashwagandha has been used to increase energy, regain strength, and help the body adapt to stress, among many other benefits. Shatavari is known to increase the quality and quantity of breast milk, maintain a healthy female reproductive system, and build strength while it nourishes you.

Imbibing these herbs in warm milk with mild spices increases their ability to nourish the deeper tissues in the body. All body types can enjoy this beverage.

Ingredients

1 cup organic milk or substitutes

1 teaspoon shatavari powder

1 teaspoon ashwagandha powder

1 pinch cardamom

1 pinch nutmeg

1 pinch cinnamon

Directions

Bring milk to a boil. Turn off the heat and add remaining ingredients. Stir well and steep covered for 5 minutes. Drizzle with honey or maple syrup and drink warm 1 hour before bed.

Both ashwagandha and shatavari are available from Banyan Botanicals and the Ayurvedic Institute. (See resources section.)

now high protein can take the back burner. Breastfeeding women typically need 2,300 to 2,500 calories per day, but that number is higher if you are underweight, nursing more than one infant, or exercising vigorously.

Postpartum women can continue with their pregnancy RDAs for the first few months, and possibly longer, depending on their health. It is wise to continue with your prenatal vitamins while you are still nursing.

You may need to pay attention to your iron intake, especially if you lost a lot of blood during birth. Essential fatty acids (especially omega-3s) are vital for a healthy nervous system, internal lubrication, hormonal balance, and preventing postpartum depression. Omega-3s are also passed to your baby through breast milk and can help with your baby's brain and eye development. Women can increase their intake of foods high in essential fatty acids, or continue with their pregnancy supplements (especially if they are experiencing postpartum depression or are susceptible to it). It is recommended for women to supplement with 300 milligrams per day of omega-3s. Make sure the company certifies that its products are free of heavy metals such as mercury, lead, and cadmium, as does Nordic Naturals. Vegetarian DHA and EPA are also available from natural sources, such as algae. See the resources section for recommended items. Refer back to chapter 3 for a list of foods high in omega-3 fatty acids.

Adequate fluid intake is also essential, since much of your body's fluids are going into your breast milk, and then into your baby. Strive to have a large glass of room temperature water every time you nurse your baby. Make a large batch of the Postpartum Nourishing Tea and sip it throughout the day. It contains herbs for increasing iron, toning the uterus, calming the nervous system, increasing milk supply, and soothing digestion.

Foods and Herbs to Increase Breast Milk

Alfalfa
Almonds
Avocado
Barley
Beets
Brown rice
Carrots
Dandelion root and leaves
Fennel
Fenugreek
Marshmallow root
Milk
Milky oats
Mochi (a Japanese food made from pounded sweet rice, available from natural food stores)
Nettle
Oatmeal
Raspberry leaf
Shatavari
Winter squash

Ayurvedic Baby Massage

Massaging babies has been an Ayurvedic practice for thousands of years. In India, babies are typically massaged throughout their first year of life, or at least for a minimum of forty days after birth. Many other traditional cultures around the world also have customs for infant massage. Since the beginning of time, this practice has been passed down from mother to daughter. Now infant massage is being rediscovered in the modern world, and scientific studies are proving that it offers a multitude of benefits.

An oil massage is food for your baby's body. It directly nourishes the baby's nervous system and skin, improving skin texture, color, and softness. It aids your baby's digestion by relieving constipation, colic, and gas. Neurological development is stimulated, and immune function is increased. Babies often sleep better and feel more relaxed, soothed, and comfortable after a massage. When infants of mothers who had postpartum depression received massage, they spent more time in active-alert and active-awake states, cried less, and had lower salivary cortisol levels (compared to infants who were rocked), which suggests that they had lower stress. The massage-therapy infants gained more weight, showed greater emotional and social improvement, and had less urinary stress, and fewer stress hormones.

Postpartum Nourishing Tea

Ingredients
1 cup nettle leaf
1 cup raspberry leaf
1 cup milky oats
½ cup fennel seeds
½ cup orange peel
¼ cup anise seeds
¼ cup ginger
¼ cup fenugreek seeds
1 quart of boiled water

Directions
Mix all the dried herbs together in a large bowl, then store in a glass jar with a lid, away from light and heat.

Place a heaping ¼ cup of mixed herbs in a quart of boiling water. Cover and let steep for 20 to 30 minutes. Strain and sweeten with honey if desired. Drink warm or at room temperature. Enjoy up to 4 cups daily.

One of the sweetest aspects of infant massage is the bond it creates between the mother or caregiver and the baby. This bonding process provides deep and crucial emotional nourishment. When the mother and baby feel loved and relaxed, it actually stimulates the production of oxytocin, the so-called love hormone, which helped bring your baby into the world and is also responsible for sexual arousal, reducing anxiety, and feeling calm and joyful. The time spent together during massage helps parents or caregivers learn about their baby's cues and how to respond to them. This can increase your confidence in your ability to care for your little one.

After your baby's umbilical cord stump has fallen off, she is ready to receive a full-body massage. You can ask the baby if she would like to receive a massage. How can a newborn tell you if she would like a massage or not? Through facial or body expressions, a particular gaze, or other nonverbal ways of communicating. Part of the subtle art of parenting is learning to tune into your baby and looking for these subtle cues. Learning how to communicate with your baby happens with time, patience, and by paying close attention. *(It is important not to massage your baby when she is congested.)*

What type of oils should you use for infant massage? Sesame or sunflower oils are good tridoshic choices. Coconut oil can be used in the summer, in warm climates, and for babies with sensitive skin. Almond and olive oils are other possibilities. Choose oils based on what you observe about your baby, cultural preferences, climate, availability, and cost. *Never use an inedible oil or mineral oil.*

Before you begin a massage, make sure the room is warm and free of drafts and dust, and that you have what you need (towels, oil, baby clothes, a diaper for after the bath, and anything else you need for yourself if you will be taking a bath with your baby). Natural and soft lighting is best. You can run a bath before the massage to add heat and moisture to your bathroom.

Here are the basic steps for giving your baby a fantastic massage:

- Warm the oil by pouring it into a plastic bottle and setting it in hot water for a few minutes. Always test the oil temperature before applying it to your baby.
- Lay your baby down on old towels that can get soiled and oiled, or place the baby on your outstretched legs. Begin with the baby facing you.
- You can sing or chant to your baby while massaging her. You can also talk to her and give her the play-by-play of the massage.
- Using gentle pressure (not too soft and not too firm), begin the massage at the head and end at the feet.
- Massage the head in a circular motion with the palm of your hand. Make sure to include all parts of the ears.
- Use extra oil on the fontanels (top of skull) in the evening to help induce sound sleep, but use care not to press on the fontanels.
- Massage the face with upward strokes—from chin to ears.
- Move down the body using circular motions around all the joints, and up and down strokes on the long bones of the arms and legs.
- Spend plenty of time, using ample oil on the belly, massaging in a clockwise direction, following the movement of the colon.

- Massage up and down on the feet, around the ankles, and tenderly pull each toe.
- Gently turn your baby over while supporting her head and massage the back with large, sweeping motions up, down, and around the entire back. Slowly move up and down the spine, from the neck to the buttocks. Massage the backs of the arms and legs and end at the feet again.
- Slowly place your baby (and maybe you too) in the warm bath when finished.

Adjusting to Your Postpartum Body and Self

The physical and emotional changes you experience during the first six to twelve weeks after giving birth, as your body attempts to return to its prepregnancy state, are almost as great as those you experience during the entire pregnancy. For some women, it takes effort to adjust to being in this stage. You may look four or six months pregnant for some time. Loving your body during this transformation is essential for a content and peaceful state of mind.

It is very important *not* to diet or rush into strong exercise programs. Your extra weight is a needed buffer for the sleeplessness and other demands on your physical and emotional body. Your pregnancy weight will come off in due time and in accordance with your constitution. I have always joked with colleagues that I can spot a Vata prakruti woman in a second when I see her holding a two-month-old baby and the woman is skinny-minny already! Pitta types will shed their extra weight with a little effort once they become active again. It can take a while for Kapha prakruti women to lose their extra weight, but with effort, patience, vigilance, and time, it will come off.

After at least six weeks, or eight if you've had a cesarean section, you can begin to get back into yoga. While postpartum is not the time for strong or intense yoga practices, simple breathing and stretching with meditation can help you keep your mind and emotions in a balanced state. Yoga is a tool to help us deal with changes, and there are many now. Working gently with the body can alleviate many common aches and pains from carrying the baby and breastfeeding. It is also an opportunity to take quiet time and do something healing for yourself.

ASANA PRACTICE

Gentle and Safe Postpartum Movement

The following is a simple asana practice to gently stretch your neck, arms, and back to help adjust to breastfeeding and carrying your baby. You will be familiar with many of the poses, which have now been adapted for your postpartum body. You can begin to say hello to your abdominal muscles again by gently engaging them with each exhale. If your lower back becomes sore quickly, then back off, and just engage your abdominal muscles half of the time during this practice.

Don't cut your time short with Viparita Karani and Shavasana. These restorative and relaxing poses will greatly help with your recovery. I have indicated a couple of places to do Kegel exercises (see page 122 for instructions) while you are in poses to help regain the muscles of your perineum. Feel free to practice them more and at other times while doing yoga. This practice can increase energy, encourage rejuvenation, and help alleviate postpartum depression.

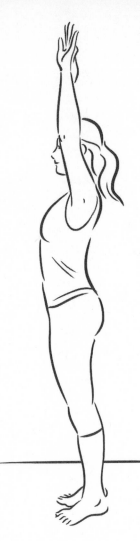

figure 23 **Tadasana**
(Mountain Pose)

1. TADASANA (MOUNTAIN POSE)
   - Stand with legs hip-width apart and your feet facing forward.
   - Feel your feet planted firmly on the ground. Your chin is gently tucked and your shoulders relaxed. Make sure your knees are soft and not locked. Keep your eyes open.
   - Place your palms on your belly and draw your breath in. Take a couple of relaxed, comfortable breaths, and then relax your arms by your side.
   - Inhale and sweep your arms out to the side and up by your ears. Very slightly arch your back as you look at your hands above your head.
   - Exhale and lower your arms back down by your sides. Lower your chin.
   - Repeat this arm movement two to three times at your own pace.

2. VIRABHADRASANA (WARRIOR POSE)
   - Stand with your legs hip-width apart and your feet facing forward.
   - Step your left foot three to four feet forward. Make sure it is a comfortable distance for you.

- Turn your right foot slightly out, so your toes point slightly to the right.
- Make sure you have enough width between your legs to feel stable and so that your hips are squared comfortably to the front. Your arms are by your sides.
- As you inhale, bend your left knee and sweep your arms by your ears. Your weight shifts forward onto your left leg. Lift your chest, gently arching your back.
- As you exhale, lower your arms and straighten your front leg, shifting your weight back.
- Repeat three times on this side and then step your feet together.
- Repeat the sequence on the other side, and then step your feet together.

3. UTTANASANA (INTENSE STRETCH POSE)
- Stand with your feet hip-width apart, facing forward.
- Inhale and lift your arms up by your ears.
- Exhale and sweep your arms out to your sides as you bend forward, slightly bending your knees, bringing your arms toward the floor with your elbows bent. As you exhale, engage your abdominal muscles by pulling them toward your spine.
- Inhale, sweep your arms back up by your sides, then overhead as you return to standing. Exhale and lower your arms back by your sides.
- Repeat two more times, then stay bent forward with your knees bent. Release your neck and let your head be heavy and relaxed. You can place your hands on your legs, on the floor, or on a rolled up blanket. Stay for a few breaths. Do a few Kegel exercises while in the forward bend.
- Press your feet into the floor and lift your upper body to come out of the pose.

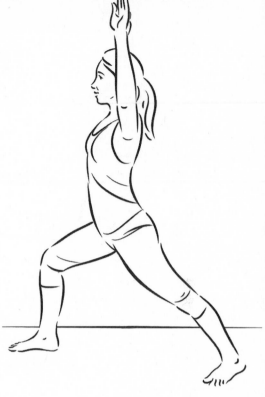

figure 24 **Virabhadrasana** (Warrior Pose)

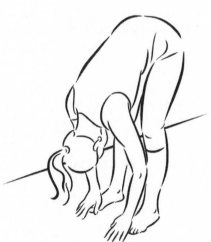

figure 25 **Uttanasana** (Intense Stretch Pose)

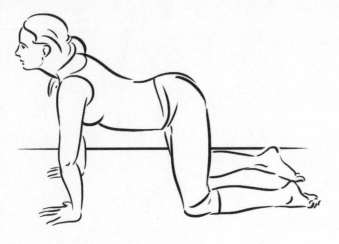

figure 26 **Cakravakasana**
(Ruddy Goose Pose)

4. CAKRAVAKASANA (RUDDY GOOSE POSE)

- Start on your hands and knees, with your hands under your shoulders and your knees under your hips or slightly wider than hip-width apart.
- On an inhalation, gently lift your chest and your head away from your belly, lifting your heart center.
- On an exhalation, pull your belly toward your spine as you round your lower back and bring your buttocks toward your heels.
- Do this three to four more times, gently linking breath and movement, and gently rocking back and forth.

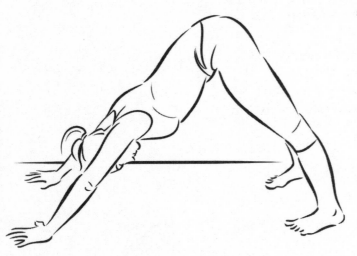

figure 27 **Adho Mukha Shvanasana** (Downward Facing Dog Pose)

5. ADHO MUKHA SHVANASANA (DOWNWARD FACING DOG POSE)

- Start on your hands and knees, with your hands directly under your shoulders and your knees directly under your hips.
- Inhale and lift your head and chest.
- Exhale, tuck your toes under, and send your buttocks up toward the sky. As you do, drop your head toward earth and straighten your arms and spine.
- Take a breath here, and then as you exhale, drop your knees back to the floor.
- Repeat the previous two steps one time.
- Inhale for a third time, and as you do, lift your head and chest. As you exhale, tuck your toes under and push your hands into the floor as your straighten your arms, sending your tailbone up to the sky.
- Now stay for three to six breaths. Keep your awareness on long and smooth breaths. While in the pose, do several Kegel exercises.
- When you are ready, drop your knees to the floor to come out of the pose.

6. ADHO MUKHA SHVANASANA TO
   URDHVA MUKHA SHVANASANA
   (DOWNWARD FACING DOG POSE
   TO UPWARD FACING DOG POSE)

   - Start on your hands and knees, with your
     hands directly under your shoulders and
     your knees directly under your hips.
   - Inhale and lift your head and chest.
     Exhale, tuck your toes under, and send
     your buttocks up toward the sky. As you
     do, drop your head toward earth and
     straighten your arms and spine. Take a full breath here.
   - Now inhale and bend your elbows, shifting your weight forward to
     your arms. Lower your body toward the floor, but not all the way.
     Keep your toes curled under and supporting you as you lift your
     chest and look upward. This is Urdhva Mukha Shvanasana.
   - Exhale and push your weight back toward your feet as you return to
     Adho Mukha Shvanasana.
   - Inhale and return to Urdhva Mukha
     Shvanasana. Engage your abdominal muscles
     as you shift your weight into Urdhva Mukha
     Shavasana.
   - Repeat several times.

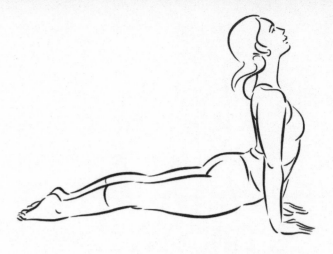

figure 28 **Urdhva Mukha Shvanasana** (Upward Facing Dog Pose)

7. PASCHIMOTTANASANA
   (STRETCH TO THE WEST POSE)

   - Sit on your buttocks, with your legs stretched
     out in front of you. You can sit on a folded
     blanket to get more length in your legs.
   - Inhale, lengthen your spine, and lift your arms up by your ears.
   - Exhale and bend forward from the hips, letting your arms land
     somewhere on your legs or feet. As you bend and exhale, pull your
     abdominal muscles toward your spine.
   - Repeat the movement sequence three more times. Then stay in the
     forward bend for five to ten breaths. Do not collapse forward. Keep
     the length in your spine; lift your head and chest with your chin
     slightly tucked.
   - Inhale to come out of the pose and relax your arms by your side.

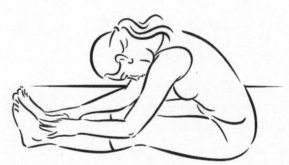

figure 29 **Paschimottanasana** (Stretch to the West Pose)

8. VIPARITA KARANI (INVERTED-DOING POSE)

- Lie on your back facing a wall.
- Slide your legs up the wall so the backs of your legs rest on the wall. You can support your uterus by placing folded blankets underneath your pelvis.
- Extend your arms outward from your body in a T position. Bend your elbows so your arms are relaxed, with your palms facing up. Tuck your shoulder blades down and back.
- Close your eyes and breathe for twelve breaths or longer. Many women enjoy staying in this pose for five minutes.
- Do several Kegel exercises while in this pose.
- To come out, press your feet into the wall and slowly roll onto your side before sitting up or moving right into Shavasana.

9. SHAVASANA (CORPSE POSE)

- Lie on your back on a blanket. Place a folded or rolled up blanket underneath your knees to relax your lower back. Cover yourself with more clothing or another blanket if you are cold.

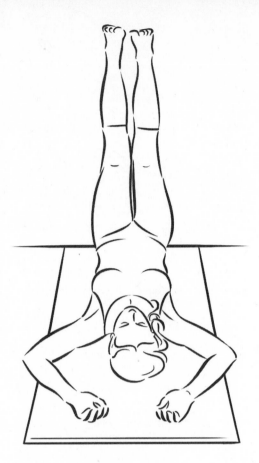

figure 30 **Viparita Karani** (Inverted-Doing Pose)

- Let your breath be natural.
- Close your eyes.
- Mentally scan your body and consciously relax any tense places. Let your whole body feel heavy and relaxed.
- Rest for five to ten minutes. Slowly roll onto your side and use your arms to get up. 🌢

BREATHING PRACTICE

Nadi Shodhana Pranayama

Nadi shodhana, or alternate-nostril breathing, is a wonderful postpartum practice because it helps to reset the flow of prana within your body and helps you return to your center. (Follow the instructions on page 134.) Do two rounds of twelve repetitions. 🌢

MEDITATION PRACTICE

The Sun as a Source of Strength

Using images of our solar system's bright star, this meditation practice can help recharge your batteries and cultivate inner strength.

- Sit comfortably. Use blankets and pillows to make yourself at ease. If you are feeling especially tired, find a restful reclining position, but make sure you're able to keep your attention on the practice and not fall asleep.
- Close your eyes and turn your attention inward. Bring your awareness to your breath. Take a few moments to observe the flow of your inhalation and exhalation. Let your breath be relaxed.
- Visualize the sun emerging on the horizon at the beginning of the day. Feel the freshness of a new day. A new beginning is in the air.
- Now visualize that sun beaming right into your heart. Feel its warmth. Feel the sun as a source of strength and radiance in your body, uplifting and energizing you.
- Let each breath bring you closer to the brightness and power of the sun. See the sun inside of you, mirroring that brightness and power. Extend this awareness to all parts of your body. Feel every cell of your body infused with this strength and energy.
- See all the solar warming colors—yellows, oranges, magentas, crimsons—shining in your heart space.
- Feel your energy revitalizing. Feel the light within yourself emerging.
- Breathe with your vision for several more breaths.
- What other images come to mind when you imagine cultivating strength and brightness within yourself? Connect with those personal images, allowing them to fill you with strength and brightness.
- Bring your awareness back to the breath moving in and out of your nose. Slowly open your eyes and take a few minutes to adjust to your surroundings before getting up. Carry this energy with you throughout your day. 🌢

SOUND PRACTICE
Surya Mantra

The sun is a remover of darkness, a nourisher of life, and a protector of health. This chant asks the sun to remove any challenges, give us strength, and guide us on our way.

- Sit in a comfortable position. You can sit cross-legged on the floor, on a cushion in Sukhasana, or in a chair.
- Let the breath lengthen the spine.
- For each of the following phrases, take a natural breath in, then exhale, reciting one line per exhale:

Om hram (om hraam)
Om hrim (om hreeem)
Om hrum (om hruum)
Om hraim (om hr-eye-m)
Om hraum (om hrouwm)
Om hrah (om hrah-hah)
Om hram, hrim, hrum, hraim, hraum, hrah
Om hram, hrim, hrum, hraim, hraum, hrah

- When finished, sit quietly for a few moments before getting up. ◗

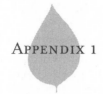

Remedies for Common Pregnancy Ailments

Let medicine be thy food, and food be thy medicine.
HIPPOCRATES

The rapid transformation of a woman's body in pregnancy is often accompanied by certain common discomforts. The magnitude of changes within your being can be felt physically, psychologically, emotionally, and sometimes, spiritually. Many simple home remedies can restore balance and lessen or relieve common conditions. Natural remedies can be more effective, less expensive, and healthier than Western medical treatments. It is best, as much as possible, to minimize your intake of drugs during pregnancy. However, these suggestions should not replace the care of your healthcare provider. *Always* consult your doctor or midwife, especially if you are unsure or uncomfortable with the recommendations.

Some of the remedies listed here have been clinically proven effective. Others are empirical and anecdotal—used by scores of women over the years. Remember, this is not a one-size-fits-all approach. One suggestion may work wonders for your pregnant friend and have no effect on you. This is why several suggestions are listed under each ailment.

Treating simple ailments at home can be fun and empowering. Diet and lifestyle are often the first line of treatment; they are simple, effective, and safe in pregnancy. In Ayurveda, commonly available herbs and spices, such as ginger and cardamom, are used as medicine, and ingesting normal amounts of cooking spices is considered safe in pregnancy. You may look at your spice cabinets with fresh eyes as many of the items discussed here may already be in your kitchen. Although some of the herbs suggested may be unfamiliar to you, let yourself be open to their healing potential. You may discover something new.

It is important to use mild herbs known to be safe in pregnancy *as directed* and in moderate amounts. Always consult with a professional herbalist, midwife, or doctor experienced in using herbs in pregnancy, and do your own research. Generally, all herbs should be avoided in the first trimester unless necessary (such as ginger or mint for morning sickness). See appendix 4 for a list of all herbs contraindicated in pregnancy, and appendix 6 for how to use essential oils safely.

The ingredients in the remedies outlined here are readily available from reliable sources in the United States. Some of these recommended items may be purchased at a local herb shop or health food store, while others may be purchased online. See the resources section for recommendations for herbal companies committed to integrity, high quality, organically grown products, heavy-metal testing, and sustainable sourcing.

Lastly, in your journey to greater self-awareness, try to see if your ailment has a hidden message or can teach you something about your current state. Listen to the language you use when describing what you are experiencing. Is something literally giving you a pain in the neck? Did you have trouble digesting a conversation you had over dinner last night? There may be an underlying emotional component. Describe the qualities of your ailment to help give you a general sense of which dosha is most involved and how to adapt your overall diet and lifestyle to remedy it. Does your ailment feel hot and sharp? If so, Pitta is involved. Do you feel dull and heavy? That is excess Kapha. Perhaps your complaint seems very erratic in nature. These are the forces of Vata at play. Or maybe, just maybe, your hidden message is simply your body craving an excuse to put your feet up and savor an afternoon cup of tea.

Anemia

Anemia is a decrease in the number of red blood cells in the body or a less than normal quantity of hemoglobin in the blood. Iron is essential for making hemoglobin, the protein in red blood cells that carries oxygen to other cells. Iron also aids protein metabolism, assists with proper muscle contraction, increases resistance to stress, ensures adequate energy, and helps the body fight infections.

During pregnancy your iron requirements increase significantly because of your growing baby and placenta. Since blood volume increases by 30 to 50 percent during pregnancy, your body needs to make more hemoglobin for the additional blood. The expanded blood volume creates a physiological anemia, so lowering levels are not always concerning. It is when levels drop below a certain value that signs of anemia may result.

Anemia in pregnancy is most commonly caused by iron deficiency, but can also develop from insufficient folic acid or B-12. Many women begin pregnancy with insufficient stores of iron, as women in general are susceptible to anemia because blood is lost every month during menses. Entering pregnancy with low iron levels can easily lead to anemia. Building up your iron stores is especially important during the last trimester to compensate for blood loss during childbirth. Keep maintaining your iron for the first few months postpartum to replenish your own red blood supply.

Iron-deficiency anemia is usually discovered from a blood test measuring your hematocrit and hemoglobin levels. You may experience symptoms linked to anemia, such as fatigue; dizziness; heart palpitations and shortness of breath; pale skin, especially in your fingernails or under your eyelids; trouble concentrating; or headaches. Your healthcare provider may suggest an iron supplement. Many of these supplements can be constipating or difficult to digest or absorb. On the contrary, many iron-rich foods, such as dried apricots and prunes, can have a laxative effect.

The remedies given here are specifically for iron-deficiency anemia. Herbs and foods can have a remarkable effect on anemia. However you choose to treat anemia, you should be monitored carefully with frequent blood tests because maternal anemia can put you at risk for preterm delivery and delivering a low birth weight baby. Anemia may also be associated with postpartum depression.

HOW TO TREAT WITH FOODS
- Eat iron-rich foods on a daily basis: beets, carrots, spinach, chard, and other dark, leafy green veggies; grapes and cherries; sunflower and pumpkin seeds; unsulfured dry fruits such as apricots, prunes, raisins, currants, figs, cherries, and dates; and seaweeds such as kelp and dulse.

Stinging Nettles: Herb Extraordinaire

In addition to being high in iron and other minerals, nettles are wonderful natural antihistamines and help to strengthen the sinuses. When I was in the second trimester of my second pregnancy, I took several freeze-dried stinging nettles capsules daily and drank nettle infusions with other herbs several times a week to counteract the effects of the Santa Fe allergy season. When I had my routine blood work at twenty-four weeks, the midwife who was working at my doctor's office told me that in her twenty years of practicing midwifery that was the first time she had seen iron levels increase during pregnancy. Thanks, nettles!

- Compote is a delicious iron-rich treat. Place 1 handful each of unsulfured dried apricots, cherries, and raisins in a saucepan, add a cinnamon stick, a thin slice of ginger, and 1 ½ cups of water. Cover and cook on medium heat for 30 to 45 minutes, stirring occasionally. When finished, remove the cinnamon and ginger. Use the compote as a topping on oatmeal or waffles, or eat by itself. Store in the refrigerator and eat within a week or two.
- Drink **fresh pressed juices**: pomegranate, carrot, and beet (and other veggies mentioned above).
- **Blackstrap molasses** is rich in iron. You can add 1 tablespoon of blackstrap molasses to 1 cup of almond milk in a glass jar with a lid. Shake and enjoy.
- If you choose to eat meat to build your iron stores, choose local, hormone-free, grass-fed, and free range animal products. Red meat and dark meat poultry are the highest iron sources.

HOW TO TREAT WITH HERBS

- The herbal supplement called **Floradix Iron and Herbs** is excellent and easily absorbable. Buy the liquid form and follow dosage instructions on the bottle. Store in the refrigerator.
- **Stinging nettle:** (1) To make a strong tea, place ½ cup nettle leaves in a teapot and fill it with 3 cups of boiling water. Steep for 1 to 2 hours and drink 2 to 4 cups each day. (2) Freeze-dried nettles in capsules are available at your local health food store. Take two to four capsules daily with food.
- **Liquid chlorophyll:** take 1 tablespoon daily added to 2 cups of water or juice.
- **Blue-green algae:** take two to six tablets a day divided out with meals.

OTHER SUGGESTIONS

- You can increase your absorption of iron by cooking in cast-iron cookware and adding a little bit of acid, in the form of lemon or orange juice, to foods.
- Take **Floradix** and iron-rich foods and herbs separate from dairy products for maximum absorption.

Back Pain

Back pain is almost inescapable during pregnancy. In preparation for birth, your body secretes hormones that loosen joints and ligaments. This softening and loosening can create physical instability, leading to back pain. As your baby grows, your weight increases and your center of gravity shifts, which can also cause back discomfort. You may compensate by leaning your torso backward, which can further strain the muscles in your lower back. Back pain can also come from poor posture, constipation, urinary tract infections, excessive standing, and exhaustion. *Always seek medical evaluation if you experience severe back pain.*

HOW TO TREAT WITH FOODS

- If you suspect constipation is involved with your back pain, read the constipation section in this appendix (page 210) and treat accordingly. Strive for at least one good bowel movement a day.

HOW TO TREAT WITH HERBS

- Massage warm oil into sore, tight, tense muscles. Add 1 to 3 drops of essential oil from frankincense or geranium to 3 tablespoons of sesame oil (or another carrier oil). Follow your massage with a warm bath with Epsom salts and essential oils such as lavender or chamomile.

OTHER SUGGESTIONS

- Perform the yoga poses Samasthiti (page 157) and Tadasana (page 109) to encourage alignment and enhance correct posture. Also practice back-strengthening yoga poses, such as Cakravakasana (see page 112).
- Exercise daily: walking, swimming, yoga.
- Perform gentle yoga poses, such as Cakravakasana (see page 112) and Tadasana (page 109) that strengthen the back and enhance correct posture.

- Wear flat, comfortable shoes with good arch support.
- Do not lift more than twenty pounds. (This can be challenging if you have a toddler.) Always bend your knees and squat when lifting heavy objects, or ask for help.
- Receive a massage if possible. Make sure the massage therapist is trained in prenatal massage, or have your partner or friend massage you while you are lying on your side.
- Use extra pillows when sleeping. This works wonders. You can place a long pillow under your belly and one between your legs when you're lying on your side. Use extra pillows under your head if necessary.
- Receive treatments from a chiropractor and/or an acupuncturist. Let them know you're pregnant.

Constipation

Constipation is defined as infrequent bowel movements that are dry, hard, and difficult to pass. This affects about half of all women during some stage of pregnancy. Constipation in pregnancy is thought to occur due to the hormone progesterone, which relaxes the smooth muscles throughout the body, especially the intestines. When the intestinal muscles relax, it can cause food and waste to move more slowly through your system. The pressure of the growing uterus on the intestines can slow things down as well. Constipation can also stem from anxiety, worry, too little physical exercise, a low-fiber diet, or from taking an iron supplement.

HOW TO TREAT WITH FOODS

- Before going to bed, drink **warm, spiced milk with ghee** for added lubrication. Warm 1 cup of milk and add a few pinches of spices (cardamom, cinnamon, ginger, and/or turmeric). Sweeten with honey or raw sugar if desired. Stir in 1 to 2 teaspoons of ghee, and drink warm.
- Increase fiber in your diet by adding extra fresh fruits and vegetables, whole grains, and beans.
- Increase good-quality oils, ghee, and dosha-appropriate oils in your diet. (See appendix 2.)
- Make **compote** out of prunes, raisins, apricots, and cherries and eat a little daily. (See instructions under "Anemia.")
- In the morning, add a couple of tablespoons of ground flax seeds or unprocessed wheat bran to hot or cold cereal.

- Consume **chia seeds,** which are naturally high in fiber. (1) Mix 2 tablespoons of chia seeds in 16 ounces of water, juice, or tea, and drink. (2) Make chia pudding by soaking ¼ cup chia seeds in 1 cup milk of your choice and ¼ cup or less of honey. Refrigerate overnight. Enjoy.

HOW TO TREAT WITH HERBS

- Take 1 teaspoon psyllium husks (also called sat isabgol) in 1 cup of warm water or milk.

OTHER SUGGESTIONS

- Exercise regularly: a minimum of thirty minutes at least three to four times per week or more. Walking, hiking, swimming, yoga, and other moderate exercise helps the intestines work by stimulating the bowels. Squatting is especially helpful.
- Drink adequate water: average eight to ten eight-ounce glasses per day. (Herbal teas, lemon water, and other hydrating beverages count too.) Half your weight in ounces is an average amount. Drink more than that when you're active or constipated. Generally, warm liquids increase elimination and cold liquids slow down elimination.
- Never delay the urge to have a bowel movement. Leave enough time to relax on the toilet and have a bowel movement.
- Place your feet on a stool while making a bowel movement.
- Do not take castor oil, triphala, other purgatives, laxative teas, or laxative pills. These are too strong during pregnancy.

My client Melissa was sixteen weeks pregnant and had constipation and lower back pain. Her diet lacked fresh fruits and vegetables, which she began to increase. She also improved circulation to her pelvis with gentle yoga asanas and swimming. At night she drank a cup of warm, spiced milk with a teaspoon of ghee. One teaspoon of ghee was too heavy for her, so she adjusted to half a teaspoon. On her first follow-up visit three weeks later she had no more constipation and her back only bothered her at the very end of her workday, when she then practiced yoga.

Edema

Edema is a condition of excess fluid accumulation in your tissues. It is normal to experience some edema in pregnancy because you are naturally retaining more water and your body is producing more blood. This extra retention of fluid is needed to soften the body, which enables it to expand as the baby develops.

Chemical changes in your blood can also cause some fluids to shift in your tissues. The enlarged uterus places pressure on the pelvic blood vessels and constricts them. This pressure slows the return of blood from your legs, causing it to pool, which forces fluid from veins into the tissues of feet and ankles and leads to swelling. Swelling can also be due to high blood pressure; lack of protein, iron, or exercise; consuming too much sodium or caffeine; poor circulation; or standing for long periods of time.

Edema can occur at any point during pregnancy, but it is most often an issue during the third trimester, particularly at the end of the day. It may be worse during the summer. This minor annoyance will go away fairly rapidly after you have your baby (within a week or two), as your body eliminates the excess fluids.

Caution: Swelling in your face or puffiness around your eyes, more than slight swelling of your hands, or excessive or sudden swelling of your feet or ankles can be signs of preeclampsia, a serious condition that requires medical supervision and *cannot* be treated at home.

HOW TO TREAT WITH FOODS

- Drink plenty of water and lemon water, which can help your body retain less water.
- Eat foods that can help release extra water: dandelion greens, cucumber, celery, watermelon, and grapefruit.
- Drink fresh juices containing cucumber, celery, apple, carrot, or beet.

HOW TO TREAT WITH HERBS

The following herbal teas are best consumed in the morning or early afternoon since they are mild diuretics and will increase the number of times you urinate. (You are probably already waking up enough times to pee during the night.)

- **Cumin, coriander, and fennel tea:** Boil 2 cups of water. Add ½ teaspoon each of whole cumin, coriander, and fennel seeds. Let the seeds steep for 5 minutes. Remove from heat, strain, and drink warm or at room temperature. Do not drink more than 2 cups daily.

- **Nettle and dandelion leaf tea:** Steep 1 teaspoon of each herb in 1 cup of boiling water for 15 minutes. Drink 1 to 2 cups daily. Dandelion leaf has a bitter taste so you may want to sweeten this tea with a touch of honey or raw sugar.

OTHER SUGGESTIONS

- Lie on your side to help relieve the increased pressure on your veins. Since the vena cava is on the right side of your body, left-sided rest works best.
- Elevate your feet so that they are at the level of your heart or slightly higher. Use bolsters, blankets, or pillows to get comfortable so you can rest for 15 to 20 minutes, a few times a day.
- Do gentle yoga such as Cakravakasana (page 112) to increase circulation.
- Wear comfortable shoes and avoid clothes that are tight around your ankles and wrists.

Fatigue

Fatigue is probably one of the earliest signs of pregnancy and is completely normal and natural. In the first few weeks of gestation, peaking progesterone levels can cause tiredness. Fatigue can also be due to low blood sugar, low blood pressure, mental stress, increased blood production, and improper digestive function.

HOW TO TREAT WITH FOODS

- Make sure you are eating adequate protein and complex carbohydrates. Do not rely on processed, sugary snacks for energy. These may give you a temporary boost but will actually deplete you in the long run. Also, all doshic types can try eating five to six small meals a day.
- **Dates** are an excellent food for increasing energy. (1) Date and milk shake: Place 3 to 5 fresh dates and 1 cup of organic milk with a pinch of cardamom in a blender. Blend until smooth. Drink in the morning or afternoon. (2) Dates soaked in ghee: Soak 10 fresh dates in a quart jar of ghee. Add 1 teaspoon of ginger and ⅛ teaspoon of cardamom, and cover for two weeks. Eat one date daily in the morning.

- **Ginger** can kindle digestive fire to make it function more effectively, which can subsequently increase energy. Chew a small slice of fresh ginger with a pinch of salt before meals.

HOW TO TREAT WITH HERBS

- **Spirulina** can be used to increase energy. Add up to 1 tablespoon of the powder to an 8-ounce smoothie or juice, or take in pill form according to the dosage instructions on the bottle.
- Infusions with **stinging nettles** can boost iron levels and nourish the adrenal glands, which can assist with combating fatigue. See the directions for stinging nettle tea under "Anemia" (page 208). Drink two to three cups per day.

OTHER SUGGESTIONS

- Rest! Go to bed early, sleep later in the morning, or take naps. Extra sleep is essential to diminish fatigue.
- Exercise. Moving your body and getting your blood and heart pumping is an easy way to increase energy. When you are tired, it can be hard to muster up the energy for exercise. Start with a fast thirty-minute walk, a few times per week.
- Yoga poses such as Adho Mukha Shvanasana (page 113) and Vrikshasana (page 157) can refresh and uplift the body and mind to help combat fatigue. Poses such as Supta Baddha Konasana (page 133) can induce a deep sense of relaxation and rejuvenation.

I was very fatigued in the first and third trimesters of my second pregnancy. I was busy with my private practice and chasing my toddler around. Drinking date shakes in the morning and getting in bed at eight o'clock when my daughter went to bed significantly alleviated my fatigue.

Headaches

Some women experience headaches in pregnancy. Headaches can occur in any stage, but tend to be most common during the first and third trimesters. In the first trimester, adjusting to hormonal surges can cause pressure in the blood vessels to change and increase blood volume, causing headaches. Third trimester headaches can be from poor posture and tension from carrying extra weight. Headaches can also be caused by lack of sleep, dehydration, stress, tension, fatigue, hunger, low blood sugar, constipation, allergies, sinus congestion, and changes in your vision. Eliminating caffeine during pregnancy can also create headaches.

About two-thirds of women who suffer from migraines (characterized by moderate to severe throbbing pain, typically on one side of the head) find that their migraines actually improve during pregnancy. However, some women find no change in their migraines, or experience them with more intensity during pregnancy.

Understanding the doshas can help to classify and treat headaches. Vata-type headaches can be caused by tension, stress, constipation, nervousness, and physical overactivity. These headaches tend to occur in the occipital (back) region of the head. Pitta-type headaches are often caused from overheating, stress, and consuming Pitta-provoking foods, which can lead to acid indigestion/hyperacidity. These headaches tend to be in the temples or temporal (side) areas. Kapha-type headaches are often caused by congestion and create sinus headaches in the frontal and nasal areas of the head. With this understanding, you can use dosha-appropriate diet and lifestyle changes.

Caution: Consult with your healthcare provider if your headache worsens or becomes persistent, and if it is accompanied by blurry vision, sudden weight gain, pain in the upper right abdomen, or swelling in the hands and face.

HOW TO TREAT WITH FOODS
- Eat well-balanced, small, and frequent meals to maintain your blood sugar. Focus on high-protein, high-carbohydrate snacks.
- Dehydration is often a causative factor in headaches. Make sure you are drinking a tall glass of room temperature water every few hours or more throughout the day. Hydrating beverages such as coconut water, herbal (non-caffeinated) teas, and electrolyte drinks can be consumed as well.
- If constipation is contributing to your headache, please read the "Constipation" section and treat it accordingly. Having at least one bowel movement a day can relieve headaches.

HOW TO TREAT WITH HERBS
- Gentle, calming herbs can relax the body and mind and reduce tension. **Chamomile, tulsi, milky oats, lemon balm, and skullcap** can all be taken as teas individually or together. Steep 2 teaspoons of herbs in 1 cup of boiling water for 10 minutes, covered. Drink hot.

OTHER SUGGESTIONS

- Get plenty of rest and relaxation.
- Practice good posture.
- Practice dosha-appropriate exercise and yoga daily to help increase oxygen in the body, combat stress, and improve digestive function, which can reduce the frequency of headaches.

FOR SINUS HEADACHES

- Apply warm compresses around your eyes and nose.
- Use a eucalyptus or peppermint oil steam. Boil water in a large pot. Add a couple drops of eucalyptus or peppermint essential oil. Drape a large towel over your head and lean over the pot. Inhale the steam for five minutes.

FOR TENSION HEADACHES

- Massage the muscles of your neck and shoulders with warm sesame oil, and then take a warm shower.
- Gently massage the top of your head and the soles of your feet with warm sesame, brahmi, or coconut oil before bedtime. You may want to place a towel on your pillow and wear socks to prevent oil stains on your linens.

FOR MIGRAINE HEADACHES

- Try Shitali Pranayama (see page 91).
- Avoid direct sunlight.
- Gently massage your scalp and the soles of your feet before bed with brahmi oil. You may want to place a towel on your pillow and wear socks to prevent oil stains on your linens.

Heartburn and Indigestion

I have never met a pregnant woman whose tummy wasn't upset at least once during her pregnancy. First trimester digestive upset is generally covered under the "Morning Sickness" section. Heartburn and indigestion are most common in the second and third trimesters. The strength of the digestive fire (agni) becomes compromised in pregnancy for a couple of reasons. One reason is that increased levels of progesterone relax the muscles in the esophagus and stomach walls, leaving the flap (lower esophageal sphincter) that separates them slightly open, which makes it easier for stomach acid to travel up the esophagus. This creates an uncomfortable burning sensation. Also, as pregnancy progresses, the growing baby can put upward pressure on the stomach, making heartburn more likely.

The good news is that these digestive upsets can be treated easily and naturally with foods, herbs, and lifestyle changes, and by avoiding causative factors. Do not consume over-the-counter antacids without speaking to your healthcare provider. Some antacids contain high levels of sodium, which can cause fluid buildup in body tissues. Some may also contain lead.

HOW TO TREAT WITH FOODS

- A Pitta-pacifying diet works wonders for alleviating heartburn. Avoid all hot, spicy, oily, and fermented foods, citrus fruits, chocolate, and coffee. (See food lists in appendix 2 for more details.)
- Increase the following in your diet: cilantro, coriander, coconut, fennel, and cardamom.
- Finish your meal with a **lassi,** a classic Indian yogurt drink, or have a little plain or vanilla yogurt with your meals. To make lassi, blend ½ cup of plain yogurt with 2 cups of water and 2 tablespoons of natural sugar. You can add a pinch of ginger or cumin powder and/or ⅛ teaspoon of rosewater.
- Be aware of improper food combinations. Generally, fruits are best eaten alone, and avoid bananas with milk.

HOW TO TREAT WITH HERBS

- **Slippery elm** is an herb that contains a high amount of mucilage, which soothes irritations in the esophagus and belly. Slippery elm lozenges are readily available at your natural foods store and can be consumed freely. Make sure the lozenges contain *only* slippery elm. In my pregnancies, I carried a box in my purse to always have on hand.
- **Slippery elm tea:** Pour 8 ounces of boiling water over 1 teaspoon of slippery elm powder. You can add a pinch of cardamom if you like. Steep for 15 minutes and drink one 8-ounce cup as needed, up to four cups a day. Sweeten with honey if desired.
- **Cumin, coriander, and fennel tea** is a classic formula for gently stoking the digestive fire and assuaging indigestion, gas, and bloating. See recipe under "Edema."

- **Chamomile tea** also helps with digestive upsets. Boil 1 cup of water, and infuse it with 1 to 2 teaspoons of chamomile flowers for 10 minutes. Strain and drink warm.

OTHER SUGGESTIONS

- Don't overeat.
- Eat several smaller meals instead of three large ones to avoid overburdening your digestive system.
- Try to eat slowly and consciously, making sure to chew your food well.
- Eat sitting up, and try to remain upright for several hours after eating.
- When experiencing acid reflux, practice the yoga pose Virasana with Arm Movements (Hero Pose, page 146).
- If lying down causes heartburn, sleep with extra pillows under your head.
- Avoid eating for emotional reasons. Indigestion can occur when food is consumed and the body is not really hungry.

Insomnia

There are many reasons why sleeping soundly is a challenge in pregnancy. Many women are excited and anxious about their pregnancy. Physical discomfort such as back pain and increased belly size can make it tough to feel comfortable in bed. Heartburn, frequent urination, and NVP can contribute as well. Rest assured that insomnia during pregnancy is normal and affects approximately 78 percent of pregnant women.

HOW TO TREAT WITH FOODS

- First, make sure you are eating adequately throughout the day. Though you should avoid eating a large, heavy, spicy meal too close to bedtime, pregnant women often need a snack before bed. Make it high-protein/high-calcium such as yogurt, almond butter on toast, or warm, spiced milk.
- **Warm, spiced milk:** Warm 1 cup of milk (whole for Vata, 2% for Pitta, and skim or milk substitutes for Kapha). Add a pinch of ginger, cinnamon, cardamom, and/or turmeric. Sweeten with honey, if desired.
- Some women also need a snack in the middle of the night; leave something by your bed, such as a banana, crackers, almonds, or whatever you are craving, as long as it will not give you indigestion.

HOW TO TREAT WITH HERBS

- Gentle herbs to relax the nervous system can help promote sound sleep. Try to drink the following teas in the evening but not within an hour of bedtime, otherwise you may wake more often to pee in the night.
- **Chamomile tea:** Steep 1 to 2 teaspoons of chamomile flowers in 8 ounces of boiling water. Cover and steep for up to 10 minutes. If you use chamomile tea bags, steep 1 large or 2 small bags in 8 ounces of boiling water. Drink warm. Sweeten with honey and milk, or milk substitute, if desired.
- **Chamomile, lemon balm, and lavender tea:** Steep ½ teaspoon of chamomile, ½ teaspoon of lemon balm, and ¼ teaspoon of lavender flowers in 1 cup of boiling water. Cover and steep for 10 minutes. Drink warm. Sweeten with honey and milk, or milk substitute, if desired.
- **Skullcap** is a great sleep aid that helps relax the nervous system and induce sleep. You can add the dried herb to any of the above teas or take 15–20 drops of the tincture added to a small amount of water, twice in the hour before bedtime or in the middle of the night when you're awake.

OTHER SUGGESTIONS

- Mild aerobic exercise at least three times a week can increase your ability to sleep well.
- Choose your evening activities wisely. Do not get on the computer or watch stimulating movies after dinner. Give yourself plenty of time to unwind before going to bed. Read an enjoyable book in the evening. It may be better for you *not* to read pregnancy books before bed.
- Give yourself a warm oil massage followed by a warm bath with several drops of lavender essential oil. See "Nurturing Practice: Warm Lavender Baths," in chapter 10 (page 108).
- Practice yoga slowly, and calming pranayama, such as shitali (page 91), or nadi shodhana (page 134), before bed.
- So Hum meditation (page 98) is helpful. Practice for 15 minutes.
- Make your bedroom a clean and uncluttered space used only for sleeping, resting, and making love. Make sure the room is a comfortable temperature and dark for sleeping.
- Receive massage from a massage therapist trained in prenatal massage.

Kathryn was having trouble sleeping at twenty-two weeks because she was constantly hungry and could not get comfortable. I suggested she eat a snack before bedtime and put another snack on her night table to have when she woke in the middle of the night, as well as make sure she had adequate pillows to support her belly, back, and neck. After a few nights of bananas at 2:00 a.m. and purchasing an extra-long pillow to put between her legs, she was sleeping soundly again.

Leg Muscle Cramps

Leg cramps are painful, involuntary muscle contractions that often occur at night in the second and third trimesters. While the exact cause is not clear, some research suggests that there is a connection between leg cramps and the buildup of lactic and pyruvic acids, which occurs as a result of impaired blood flow in the legs. Leg cramps may indicate that you need more minerals. Muscles can spasm due to insufficient calcium or magnesium.

Caution: Persistent leg pain with local heat, redness, and swelling can be from phlebitis (inflammation of veins) or deep vein thrombosis (DVT blood clot). Contact your healthcare provider in this case.

HOW TO TREAT WITH FOODS

- Increase your intake of foods rich in minerals (especially calcium and magnesium) such as sea vegetables, dark leafy greens, yogurt, milk, nuts, and seeds (especially sesame seeds).
- You may want to try a calcium-magnesium supplement if your cramping is extreme. Make sure the ratio is two to one of calcium to magnesium.
- Insufficient salt intake can cause muscle cramps. Cook with sea salt or other salt alternatives such as tamari, Bragg Liquid Aminos, or Herbamare.
- Consume foods high in potassium: bananas, dried apricots, beets, cantaloupes, lima beans, winter squash, spinach, and raisins.

HOW TO TREAT WITH HERBS

- Enjoy the minerals in Nourishing Pregnancy Tea (pages 66–67).

OTHER SUGGESTIONS

- Stay active. Regular physical activity may prevent leg cramps.

- Wear comfortable shoes and avoid standing for long periods of time, if possible.
- Elevate your legs several times throughout the day.
- Make sure you are consuming enough fluids throughout the day.
- Stretching can help prevent cramps and be used during cramps. Before you go to bed, slowly and calmly practice Virabhadrasana (Warrior Pose, page 110) and Prasarita Padottanasana (Expanded Leg Stretch, page 111) to gently stretch your leg muscles.
- Rotate your ankles to increase circulation.
- Before bedtime, take a warm bath with a few handfuls of Epsom salts to relax tired muscles.
- Massage your calves and thighs daily with oil. *Do not massage over varicose veins or if you are experiencing leg pain with swelling.*

Morning Sickness

Morning sickness is a telltale sign of pregnancy, beginning around six weeks, and can last until the fourteenth week. It is rare for it to last the entire pregnancy. Morning sickness is a catchall term for nausea, queasiness, and vomiting (referred to as NVP—nausea and vomiting in pregnancy). However, it can strike at any time—day or night.

It is important to acknowledge that these symptoms are completely normal in pregnancy. Please reread pages 87–88 for more information, including the Ayurvedic perspective, on morning sickness.

Caution: Persistent or repeated vomiting in pregnancy can be a medical problem that should be addressed by your doctor or midwife.

HOW TO TREAT WITH FOODS

- Place a light snack by your bed to begin the day with a little food— some crackers, a handful of almonds, or toast.
- Frequent high-protein snacks or many small meals throughout the day and night will prevent the stomach from becoming empty and acidic. Many women find relief from snacking on lightly salted crackers throughout the day.
- Eat every two hours to help keep down the acidity, regulate the blood sugar, and keep nausea at bay.
- Coconut water works wonderfully to settle the stomach. You can drink it plain or add a teaspoon of lemon juice and take small sips every fifteen minutes.

- In general, a woman should eat foods and drinks that she is craving, because if she is craving them, she will probably not reject them.

HOW TO TREAT WITH HERBS

- **Ginger** in all forms works very well for many women. **Caution:** Do not exceed the following recommended dosages, and only take ginger with your doctor or midwife's approval if you have a history of miscarriage.
  - Drink ginger ale.
  - Cook with fresh ginger.
  - Drink **ginger tea**. Steep 2 teaspoons of freshly grated ginger in 2 cups of boiling water for 10 minutes. You can strain the tea if you like, or let the ginger settle to the bottom. Add honey if desired, and sip throughout the day. Do not drink more than 2 cups daily.
  - Nibble on ginger candies and small pieces of crystallized ginger throughout your day. The daily dose is up to 1 gram. Both crystallized ginger and candies are easy to carry with you. However, make sure to brush and floss your teeth well after consuming sugar throughout your day.
  - Take two ginger capsules every few hours, but no more than ten daily.
- **Shatavari** is a wonderful herb that can settle the stomach due to its demulcent properties. It is also building and nourishing in pregnancy. **Caution:** Do not take shatavari if you are prone to fibrocystic changes in the breasts, uterine fibroids, or other symptoms related to estrogen dominance.
  - You can take shatavari in tablets. Take one to two tablets, once or twice daily, or as directed by your healthcare practitioner.
  - You can make a **milk decoction with shatavari and mild spices**. Bring 1 cup of milk to a boil in a small saucepan. Turn off the heat and stir in 1 teaspoon of shatavari and ⅛ teaspoon each of cardamom and ginger. Cover and steep for 10 to 15 minutes. Sweeten with honey if desired, and drink while still warm. It is best before bedtime.
- **Peppermint** helps some women. You can drink peppermint tea, eat peppermint candies, chew gum, or smell the essential oil.

OTHER SUGGESTIONS

- Take a walk in the fresh air.

- Avoid foods and smells that nauseate you.
- Shitali pranayama (see page 91) has a lovely cooling and calming effect on the body and mind, which makes it very useful to relieve stress, reduce Pitta, and settle the stomach.
- Get plenty of rest and relaxation, but don't lie down right after eating.

Marcia was having awful morning sickness at eight weeks. We discussed diet, herbal, and lifestyle changes she could make. After four days of making nightly milk decoctions with shatavari and cardamom, she called me, totally astounded that the morning sickness was gone.

Skin Troubles

Some women experience the best skin of their lives while pregnant. A radiant glow on a pregnant woman's face is characteristic of the changes happening, especially increased blood flow. Many women also experience skin issues such as dry, itchy skin. This most often occurs on the regions that stretch to accommodate the baby's growth. Stress can also manifest as itchy skin.

Caution: If itchy skin progressively worsens or is persistent, you should consult with your healthcare provider.

HOW TO TREAT WITH FOODS

- Eat plenty of healthy fats, such as good-quality oils, avocados, nuts, seeds, and possibly fish, such as salmon.
- Consume a minimal intake of salt, saturated fats, and fried foods.
- Drink plenty of pure, room-temperature water. (See page 211 for recommended amount.)
- Eat plenty of fresh vegetables and fruits daily.

HOW TO TREAT WITH HERBS

- Lovingly massage herbal oil into your entire body daily. Revisit the abhyanga instructions on how to do self-massage and see appendix 5 for instructions on how to make an herbal oil.
- Massage plain coconut oil into the skin. This will soften, nourish, and hydrate the skin, and reduce itching.

OTHER SUGGESTIONS

- Avoid hot showers, which can dry out your skin and make itching worse.
- Avoid using soap on your entire body, and use only a natural, mild soap on areas that can harbor bacteria and odor, such as the armpits and feet.
- Try not to scratch! Just keep massaging oils into the skin.
- Exercise daily to increase circulation and create healthy blood flow to your skin.
- Supplementing with the essential fatty acids (EFAs) that naturally occur in fish oils and algae can improve skin health and reduce inflammation. Purchase a supplement especially for pregnant women, such as Nordic Naturals' Prenatal DHA or Algae Omega. (See resources section for more information.)

Lucia was experiencing very dry, itchy skin in her third trimester. She bought a large bottle of coconut oil and left it in her shower so she could do abhyanga daily. Within a week her skin became soft, hydrated, and smooth.

Sore Breasts

Swollen and tender breasts are a very common early sign of pregnancy. Hormonal changes during pregnancy cause increased blood flow and changes in the breast tissue, naturally resulting in larger breasts. Breasts may be sore to the touch, swollen, tingly, and especially sensitive. Some women notice changes in their breasts as early as one or two weeks after conception. This typically goes away, but some women's breasts do feel sensitive throughout the course of pregnancy.

HOW TO TREAT WITH HERBS

- Gently massage your breasts daily from the periphery to the center.
- For tenderness in early pregnancy, try Dr. Aviva Romm's sore breast massage oil recipe. To 3 ounces of sweet almond oil, add ½ ounce each of St. John's wort and arnica oils. Also add ½ teaspoon each lavender essential oil, rosemary essential oil, and rose geranium essential oil.

OTHER SUGGESTIONS

- Purchase a good supportive bra that is the correct size. Ask for help fitting if needed.
- Take a warm bath and make sure the water covers your breasts, to relieve tenderness and discomfort.

Food Guidelines

These food lists are guidelines to give you general ideas of what is best for each dosha. Individual modifications often need to be made. Moderation is the key.

Please note:

* Indicates foods that should only be consumed occasionally.

† Indicates foods that are okay in moderation when they are well cooked, well spiced, and prepared with adequate quality oils or ghee.

Fruits to Favor

VATA	PITTA	KAPHA
Sweet Fruits	**Sweet Fruits**	**Astringent Fruits**
apples (cooked)	apples (sweet)	apples (raw and cooked)
apricots	apricots (sweet)	apricots
avocados	avocados	berries (all)
bananas	berries (sweet)	cherries
berries (all)	coconut	cranberries
cherries	dates	dried fruits
coconut	figs (fresh)	figs (dry)
dates (fresh)	grapes (red and purple)	grapes*
figs (fresh)	kiwi*	kiwi*
grapefruit	limes	lemons
grapes	mangoes	limes*
kiwi	melon	mangoes
lemons	oranges (sweet)*	peaches
limes	pears	pears
mangoes	pineapple (sweet)	persimmons
melon	plums (sweet)	pomegranate
oranges	pomegranate	prunes
papaya	prunes	quince
peaches	quince*	raisins
pineapple	raisins	strawberries*
plums	strawberries*	tangerines
prunes (soaked)	watermelon	
raisins (soaked)		
rhubarb		
tangerines		

Note: For optimal digestion, consume fruits and fruit juices on an empty stomach at least twenty minutes before a meal.

Fruits to Avoid

VATA	PITTA	KAPHA
Dried Fruits	**Sour Fruits**	**Sweet and Sour Fruits**
apples (raw)	apples (sour)	avocados
cranberries	apricots (sour)	bananas
dates (dry)	bananas	coconuts
figs (dry)	berries (sour)	dates
pears	cherries (sour)	figs (fresh)
persimmons	cranberries	grapefruit
pomegranates	grapefruit	kiwi
prunes (dry)	grapes (green)	mangoes
quince	lemons	melon
raisins (dry)	oranges (sour)	oranges
watermelon	papaya	papaya
	peaches	pineapple
	persimmons	plums
	plums (sour)	rhubarb
	rhubarb	watermelon

Vegetables to Favor

VATA	PITTA	KAPHA
Cooked Veggies	**Sweet and Bitter Veggies**	**Raw, Pungent, and Bitter Veggies**
artichokes	artichokes	artichokes
asparagus	asparagus	asparagus
beets	beets (cooked)	beets and beet greens
broccoli †	broccoli	broccoli
carrots	Brussels sprouts	Brussels sprouts
cauliflower (cooked) †	burdock root	burdock root
corn (sweet and fresh)*	cabbage	cabbage
cucumbers	carrots*	carrots
daikon radishes	cauliflower	cauliflower
fennel	celery	celery
garlic	corn (sweet and fresh)*	corn
green beans	cucumbers	daikon radish
kale †	dandelion greens	eggplant
leafy greens †	fennel	fennel
leeks	green beans	garlic
lettuce*	jicama	green beans
okra	kale	kale
olives	leafy greens	kohlrabi
onions (cooked)	leeks	leafy greens
parsnips	lettuce	leeks mushrooms
peas	mushrooms*	lettuce
potatoes (sweet)	okra	okra
radishes	olives (black)	onions
rutabaga	onions (cooked)	parsley
summer squash	parsley (small amounts)	parsnips*
winter squash	parsnips	peas
	peas	peppers
	peppers (sweet)	radishes
	potatoes (sweet and white)	spinach
	rutabaga	tomatoes (cooked)
	spinach*	turnips and turnip greens
	summer squash	
	winter squash	

Vegetables to Avoid

VATA	PITTA	KAPHA
Raw, Frozen, or Dried Veggies	**Pungent Veggies**	**Sweet and Juicy Veggies**
beet greens	beets and beet greens (raw)	cucumbers
Brussels sprouts	chilies (green and red)	mushrooms
burdock root	daikon radish	olives (black and green)
cabbage	eggplant	rutabaga
cauliflower	garlic	summer squash
celery	olives (green)	sweet potatoes
dandelion greens	onions (raw)	tomatoes (raw)
eggplant	peppers (hot)	winter squash
kohlrabi	radishes	
mushrooms	tomatoes	
onions (raw)	turnips and turnip greens	
peas (raw)		
peppers		
potatoes (white)		
tomatoes		
turnips		
sprouts		

Grains to Favor

VATA	PITTA	KAPHA
amaranth*	barley	barley
barley*	cereal (dry)	buckwheat
buckwheat*	couscous	cereal (cold, dry, or puffed)
oats (cooked)	granola	corn
quinoa	oat bran	couscous
rice (all types)	quinoa	granola
spelt	rice (all types; basmati is best)	millet
wheat (regular and sprouted)	spelt	oat bran
	wheat (regular and sprouted)	quinoa
		rice (basmati and wild)
		rye
		spelt*
		sprouted wheat
		tapioca

Grains to Avoid

VATA	PITTA	KAPHA
cereal (cold, dry, or puffed)	amaranth	oats (cooked)
corn	buckwheat	rice (brown and white)
couscous	corn	wheat
granola	millet	
millet	oats (dry)	
oats (dry)	rye	
oat bran		
rye		
tapioca		

Beans and Legumes to Favor

VATA	PITTA	KAPHA
aduki beans	aduki beans	aduki beans
black beans †	black beans	black beans
lentils (brown) †	black-eyed peas	black-eyed peas
lentils (red)	chickpeas	chickpeas
mung beans (whole and split)	kidney beans	lentils (red and brown)
pinto beans †	lentils (brown)	lima beans
tempeh †	lentils (red)*	mung beans (whole and split)
tofu †	lima beans	navy beans
	mung beans (whole and split)	pinto beans
	navy beans	split peas
	pinto beans	tempeh*
	soybeans	tofu (warm)*
	split peas	white beans*
	tempeh*	
	tofu	
	white beans	

Beans and Legumes to Avoid

VATA	PITTA	KAPHA
black-eyed peas		kidney beans
chickpeas		soy beans
kidney beans		tofu (cold)
navy beans		
soybeans		
split peas		
white beans		

Note to all doshic types: Organic, non-GMO soybeans in the form of edamame, tofu, tempeh, and miso are the best choices for soy products, especially when prepared warm with dosha-appropriate spices. All doshic types should avoid or minimize highly processed soy products.

Nuts and Seeds to Favor

VATA	PITTA	KAPHA
In moderation:	almonds (soaked and peeled)	almonds (soaked and peeled)*
almonds	flax seeds	chia seeds
brazil nuts	popcorn	flax seeds*
cashews	psyllium	popcorn
chia seeds	pumpkin seeds	pumpkin seeds*
filberts	sesame seeds*	sesame seeds*
flax seeds	sunflower seeds	sunflower seeds*
hazelnuts		
macadamia nuts		
peanuts		
pecans		
pine nuts		
pistachios		
psyllium*		
pumpkin seeds		
sesame seeds		
sunflower seeds		
walnuts		

Nuts and Seeds to Avoid

VATA	PITTA	KAPHA
popcorn	Brazil nuts	Brazil nuts
	cashews	cashews
	chia seeds	chia seeds
	filberts	filberts
	hazelnuts	hazelnuts
	macadamia nuts	macadamia nuts
	peanuts	peanuts
	pecans	pecans
	pine nuts	pine nuts
	pistachios	pistachios
	walnuts	walnuts

Dairy Products to Favor

VATA	PITTA	KAPHA
butter	butter (unsalted)	buttermilk*
buttermilk	cheese (soft)	cottage cheese*
cheese (hard)*	cottage cheese	ghee*
cheese (soft)	cow milk	goat cheese*
cottage cheese	ghee	goat milk
cow milk	goat cheese	yogurt (fresh, spiced, and diluted)*
ghee	goat milk	
goat cheese	ice cream*	
goat milk	yogurt (fresh and diluted)	
sour cream*		
yogurt (fresh and spiced)		

Dairy Products to Avoid

VATA	PITTA	KAPHA
ice cream	butter (salted)	butter (salted and unsalted)
powdered milk (goat and cow)	buttermilk	cheese (soft and hard)
yogurt (frozen or plain)	cheese (hard)	cow milk
	sour cream	ice cream
	yogurt (frozen or plain)	sour cream
		yogurt (frozen or plain)

Animal Protein to Favor

VATA	PITTA	KAPHA
beef	buffalo	chicken (white)
buffalo	chicken (white)	eggs
chicken (dark and white)	egg whites	fish (freshwater)
eggs	fish (freshwater)	rabbit
fish (sea and freshwater)	rabbit	salmon*
salmon	salmon*	shrimp
sardines	shrimp*	turkey (white)
shrimp	turkey (white)	venison
tuna	venison	
turkey (white and dark)		

Animal Protein to Avoid

VATA	PITTA	KAPHA
lamb	beef	beef
pork	chicken (dark)	buffalo
rabbit	egg yokes	chicken (dark)
venison	fish (sea)	fish (sea)
	lamb	lamb
	pork	pork
	sardines	sardines
	tuna fish	tuna fish
	turkey (dark)	turkey (dark)

Oils to Favor

VATA	PITTA	KAPHA
All oils are generally fine	avocado*	**In small amounts:**
almond	coconut	corn
ghee	flax	ghee*
mustard	ghee	olive*
olive	olive	mustard
sesame	safflower*	safflower
	soy	sunflower
	sunflower	
	walnut	

Oils to Avoid

VATA	PITTA	KAPHA
	almond	avocado
	corn	coconut
	mustard	sesame
	sesame (dark)	soy
		walnut

Sweeteners to Favor

VATA	PITTA	KAPHA
barley malt	barley malt	fruit juice concentrates
brown rice syrup	brown rice syrup	honey
fructose	fructose	maple syrup*
fruit juice concentrates	fruit juice concentrates	
honey	honey*	
jaggery	maple syrup	
maple syrup	sucanat	
molasses	turbinado sugar	
sucanat		
turbinado sugar		

Sweeteners to Avoid

VATA	PITTA	KAPHA
white sugar	jaggery	barley malt
	molasses	brown rice syrup
	white sugar	fructose
		jaggery
		sucanat
		turbinado sugar
		white sugar

Beverages to Favor

VATA		PITTA		KAPHA	
almond milk	grapefruit juice	almond milk*	grape juice	aloe vera juice	grape juice
aloe vera juice	lemonade	aloe vera juice	mango juice	apple cider	mango juice
apple cider	mango juice	apple juice	miso broth*	apple juice*	peach nectar
apricot juice	milk (warm and spiced)	apricot juice	orange juice*	apricot juice	pear juice
beer*		beer*	peach nectar	berry juice	pineapple juice*
berry juice (all but cranberry)	miso broth	berry juice	pear juice	black tea	pomegranate juice
	orange juice	black tea*	pomegranate juice	carrot juice	
carrot juice	papaya juice	cherry juice		cherry juice	prune juice
cherry juice	peach nectar	cold dairy drinks	prune juice	cranberry juice	soy milk (warm and spiced)
grain coffee drinks	rice milk	grain coffee drinks	rice milk	grain coffee drinks	wine (dry; red or white)*
grape juice	soy milk (warm and spiced)*		soy milk		
	wine (white)*		wine (white and dry)*		

Herbal Teas:

ajwan	fennel
bancha	fenugreek
basil	ginger
catnip	hawthorn
chai (decaffeinated)	kukicha
chamomile	lavender
cinnamon	lemongrass
cloves	licorice
elder flowers	marshmallow
eucalyptus	nettle*
	oat straw
	orange peel

Herbal Teas:

alfalfa	jasmine
bancha	kukicha
barley	lavender
basil*	lemon balm
blackberry	lemongrass
burdock	licorice
catnip	marshmallow
chai	nettle
chamomile	oat straw
chrysanthemum	passion flower
cinnamon*	peppermint
dandelion	raspberry leaf
elder	red clover
fennel	rose flowers
ginger (fresh only)	rosehips*
	sarsaparilla
hibiscus	spearmint
hops	violet
	wintergreen
	yarrow

Herbal Teas:

ajwan	hibiscus
alfalfa	hops
bancha	hyssop
barley	jasmine
basil	kukicha
blackberry	lavender
burdock	lemon balm
catnip	lemongrass
chai	nettle
chamomile	oat straw*
chicory	orange peel
chrysanthemum	osha
cinnamon	passion flower
cloves	peppermint
corn silk	raspberry leaf
dandelion	red clover
elder flowers	rose flowers
eucalyptus	rosehips*
fennel*	sage
fenugreek	sarsaparilla*
ginger	sassafras
hawthorn	spearmint
	wintergreen
	yarrow

Beverages to Avoid

VATA		PITTA		KAPHA	
apple juice	cranberry juice	apple cider	hard alcohol	almond milk	hard alcohol
black tea	hard alcohol	caffeinated drinks	lemonade	beer	lemonade
caffeinated drinks	ice cold drinks	carbonated drinks	papaya juice	caffeinated drinks	miso broth
carbonated drinks	pear juice	carrot juice	pineapple juice	carbonated drinks	orange juice
coffee	pomegranate juice	coffee	red and sweet wines	coffee	papaya juice
cold dairy drinks	red wine	cranberry juice	tomato juice	cold dairy drinks	rice milk
	soy milk (cold)	grapefruit juice		grapefruit juice	soy milk (cold)
	tomato juice				tomato juice
					wine (sweet)

Herbal Teas:

alfalfa	dandelion	ajwan	hawthorn	licorice	
barley	hibiscus	cloves	hyssop	marshmallow	
blackberry	jasmine	eucalyptus	osha		
burdock	red clover	fenugreek	red zinger		
chrysanthemum	red zinger	ginger (dry)	sage		
	yarrow		sassafras		

Spices to Favor

VATA		PITTA		KAPHA	
ajwan	mint	basil (fresh)	mint	ajwan	marjoram
allspice	mustard seeds	black pepper*	orange peel*	allspice	mint
anise	nutmeg	caraway*	parsley	anise	mustard seeds
asafoetida (hing)	orange peel	cardamom*	peppermint	asafoetida (hing)	nutmeg
basil	oregano	cinnamon*	rosemary*	basil	orange peel
bay leaf	paprika	coriander	saffron	bay leaf	oregano
black pepper	parsley	cumin	spearmint	black pepper	paprika
caraway	peppermint	dill	tarragon*	caraway	parsley
cardamom	poppy seeds	fennel	turmeric	cardamom	peppermint
cayenne*	rosemary	ginger (fresh)	vanilla	cayenne*	poppy seeds
cinnamon	saffron		wintergreen	cinnamon	rosemary
cloves	salt			cloves	saffron
coriander	savory			coriander	savory
cumin	spearmint			cumin	spearmint
dill	star anise			dill	star anise
fennel	tarragon			fennel*	tarragon
fenugreek*	thyme			fenugreek	thyme
garlic	turmeric			garlic	turmeric
ginger	vanilla			ginger	vanilla*
marjoram	wintergreen				wintergreen

Spices to Avoid

VATA		PITTA		KAPHA	
		ajwan	marjoram	salt	
		allspice	mustard seeds		
		anise	nutmeg		
		asafoetida (hing)	oregano		
		basil (dried)	paprika		
		bay leaf	poppy seeds		
		cayenne	sage		
		cloves	salt		
		fenugreek	savory		
		garlic	star anise		
		ginger (dried)	thyme		

Condiments to Favor

VATA	PITTA	KAPHA
black pepper	cilantro	black pepper
chili peppers*	coconut	chili peppers
cilantro*	dulse	cilantro
coconut	gomasio*	gomasio*
dulse	hijiki	horseradish
gomasio	kombu	ketchup*
hijiki	lime	kombu*
horseradish	mango chutney	lemon
kelp	mint leaves	mango chutney (spicy)
ketchup	seaweed*	mint leaves
kombu	sesame seeds*	mustard
lemon	soy sauce/tamari*	onions
lime	sprouts	radish
mango chutney (sweet or spicy)		scallions
mayonnaise		seaweed*
mint leaves*		sesame seeds*
mustard		sprouts
onions (cooked)		
pickles		
salt		
scallions		
seaweed		
sesame seeds		
soy sauce/tamari		
vinegar		

Condiments to Avoid

VATA	PITTA	KAPHA
onions (raw)	black pepper	coconut
sprouts	chili peppers	dulse
	horseradish	hijiki
	kelp	kelp
	ketchup	lime
	lemon	mango chutney (sweet)
	mayonnaise	mayonnaise
	mustard	pickles
	onions (raw)	salt
	pickles	soy sauce/tamari
	radish	vinegar
	salt	

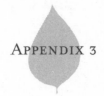

APPENDIX 3

Recipes

The following recipes feature essential prenatal nutrients in delicious, ojas-building creations. Whole grains, fresh vegetables and fruits, quality protein, healthy fats, and digestion-enhancing spices are the foundation, and minimally processed foods are the primary ingredients. The recipes are generally tridoshic (good for all types), and in the notes, I've included information on how to tailor the recipes for each type.

Organically Grown Food

While you are grocery shopping, keep in mind that organic fruits and vegetables (and dairy and meats) are safer for everyone, especially pregnant women and young children. It has been proven that residues from pesticide and chemical fertilizers can create a host of possible health problems from asthma to tumors to ADHD to cancers. However, organic groceries are more expensive and not always available. The Environmental Working Group analyzes the US Department of Agriculture's data about pesticide residue, and ranks foods based on how much or little pesticide residue they have. Its "Dirty Dozen" and "Clean Fifteen" are annually updated lists of produce with the highest and lowest pesticide residues, respectively. Here are its lists from 2012. More information and updated lists are available from the group's website, listed in the resources section.

THE DIRTY DOZEN (PLUS)

These fruits and vegetables have the highest pesticide residues. Buy organic items on this list or do not buy them at all.

1. Apples
2. Celery
3. Sweet bell peppers
4. Peaches
5. Strawberries
6. Nectarines (imported)
7. Grapes
8. Spinach
9. Lettuce
10. Cucumbers
11. Blueberries, domestic
12. Potatoes
† Green beans
† Kale/leafy greens

THE CLEAN FIFTEEN

These items have the lowest pesticide residues. You can buy these conventionally grown, without worrying about pesticide residues, if organics aren't available or are too expensive.

1. Onions
2. Sweet corn
3. Pineapples
4. Avocados
5. Cabbage
6. Sweet peas
7. Asparagus
8. Mangoes
9. Eggplant
10. Kiwi
11. Cantaloupe (domestic)
12. Sweet potatoes
13. Grapefruit
14. Watermelon
15. Mushrooms

Breakfast

COCONUT-ALMOND OATMEAL WITH MILK

Serves 4

Ingredients

1 cup rolled oats

1 cup milk

1 cup water

½ cup unsulfured dried dates, cherries, or Turkish apricots, chopped

½ teaspoon cinnamon

½ teaspoon cardamom

½ cup unsweetened shredded coconut

1 teaspoon ghee (optional)

¼ cup almond slivers or soaked and peeled almonds, chopped

Maple syrup and milk to taste

Directions

Combine rolled oats, milk, water, and dried fruit in a small saucepan and bring to a boil. Reduce heat to low; cover and simmer for 5 to 10 minutes. Add extra water or milk if you desire a thinner consistency.

Add cinnamon and cardamom and stir well.

While the oats are cooking, roast the coconut in a dry skillet on medium-high heat until slightly brown.

When the oatmeal is done, remove from heat and stir in the ghee.

Serve in individual bowls and top with almonds, toasted coconut, maple syrup, and milk of your choice.

Notes: This warm, nourishing breakfast gives you a hearty start to the day. Oats are an ideal breakfast grain since they are easier to digest than wheat or corn. Oats, combined with the almonds and milk, build ojas. Cinnamon and cardamom lighten

How to Make Ghee

Ghee is butter that has been clarified, which eliminates the hard-to-digest, cholesterol-forming milk solids. Making your own ghee is simple and much less expensive than buying it from a store. Once you try this recipe, you probably won't buy ghee again. If you make ghee on the full moon, all the juicy, bright lunar energy infuses it and increases its potency. While making ghee, chant or sing songs that make you happy.

Ingredients

1 pound unsalted organic butter

Cheesecloth

Clean and completely dry glass jar with a lid

Directions

Cook the butter in a medium-sized heavy saucepan on medium-low heat for approximately 15 to 20 minutes. The butter will bubble, and foam will rise to the surface. Do not stir. Watch carefully and avoid burning.

Milk solids will collect at the bottom of the pan toward the end of the cooking time. The ghee is finished when it is clear, quiet, and golden.

Remove from the heat and let cool for a few minutes before straining with cheesecloth into your jar. Makes 2 cups.

Store at room temperature. Ghee will keep indefinitely at room temperature if it does not become contaminated with food particles and water. Always use a clean spoon or knife when using.

the oats and milk, making them more digestible and less mucous forming. Hot cereal with milk is purported to lubricate the body and make it soft and supple. For a gluten-free version, buy oats that are labeled "gluten-free," or prepare the rice cereal on page 167.

Almonds are loaded with important minerals (including copper, manganese, magnesium, selenium, zinc, potassium, and calcium), vitamin E, healthy fats, and a small dose of protein. You can either soak them overnight in water and slide the skins off in the morning and chop, or buy them dry toasted and slivered (which usually do not have the skins on). As a busy mom, I have found many shortcuts that don't skimp on nutrition. Doing the prep work yourself ensures freshness, but when time is short it's better to take almonds from a package than to skip eating them altogether. You can use walnuts instead of almonds for a little variety. Dried fruits are high in iron and vitamin C.

Use almond milk if cow milk does not agree with you. This recipe is great for Vata and Pitta types. Kapha types can enjoy it occasionally, increasing the spices by ¼ teaspoon each, omitting the coconut and ghee, and making sure to use low- or nonfat milk.

SPINACH-LEEK FRITTATA WITH BASIL AND GOAT CHEESE
Serves 4

Ingredients
1 medium leek
3 cups fresh spinach, chopped
2 tablespoons ghee or butter
4 large eggs, plus 4 large egg whites
2 tablespoons fresh basil, chopped
2 tablespoons soft goat cheese (chèvre)
½ teaspoon sea salt

Directions
Preheat oven to 325°F.

Rinse leek well and slice finely. Wash spinach, remove any long stems, and chop finely.

Heat 1 tablespoon of ghee over medium heat in a 10-inch, ovenproof pan. When the ghee is melted, add the leek.

While the leek is cooking, mix the eggs and egg whites in a medium bowl, and whisk. Add the basil to the egg mixture.

When the leek is soft, add ½ teaspoon sea salt and the spinach. Cook for a minute or two, until the spinach is wilted. Add the remaining tablespoon of ghee and incorporate fully with the ingredients in the pan.

Turn the heat to low and add the egg mixture. Crumble the goat cheese on top and cook on low for 5 minutes, or until the edges of the eggs begin to set.

Transfer to the oven and bake uncovered for 15 to 20 minutes, until the frittata is firm and golden.

Serve warm accompanied by whole grain toast with ghee, or roasted sweet potatoes.

Notes: This scrumptious, high-protein breakfast makes a fantastic Sunday morning brunch or a satisfying meal any time of day. Eggs contain over twelve vitamins and minerals, including choline, which promotes your baby's overall growth and brain health, while helping prevent neural tube defects. Each egg has about 6 grams of protein: 3 grams in the yolk and 3 grams in the white.

Look for eggs naturally loaded with DHA, a type of omega-3 fatty acid that is essential for the fetus's brain development and eye formation. Spinach is a powerhouse of essential pregnancy nutrients: folic acid, iron, vitamin A, and calcium. A bag of prewashed baby spinach is a great time-saver that can be used here. Fresh basil subtly permeates the eggs, but if you cannot find it fresh use dried basil or pesto. Leeks have a mild, sweet flavor that creates a rich, buttery texture when slowly sautéed. Sometimes leeks can harbor dirt and sand in between their layers. Slice thinly and then soak in a bowl of cold water for a few minutes to allow the grit to sink to the bottom. Goat cheese adds a creamy, calcium-rich addition that blends well with the other ingredients.

High Pitta and Kapha types who are sensitive to whole eggs (either to their cholesterol or heaviness) can occasionally enjoy this dish or prepare it with egg whites. Kapha types can also omit the cheese and add some freshly ground black pepper.

DELECTABLE GRANOLA

Dry Ingredients
3 cups rolled oats
½ cup shredded unsweetened coconut
2 teaspoons wheat flour or spelt flour
½ teaspoon sea salt

2 tablespoons ground cinnamon

½ teaspoon ground ginger

½ cup sunflower seeds

½ cup chopped almonds

½ cup chopped walnuts

2 tablespoons sesame seeds

1 cup unsulfured dried fruit (apricots, cherries, raisins, and/or dates), rinsed and chopped

Wet Ingredients

¼ cup warmed ghee or light vegetable oil such as sunflower

½ cup pure maple syrup

1 tablespoon vanilla extract

Directions

Preheat oven to 325°F.

Combine the oats, coconut, flour, salt, cinnamon, and ginger in a large bowl and mix well. In another bowl, mix the sunflower seeds, almonds, walnuts, and sesame seeds.

Stir all the wet ingredients into the oat mixture, ensuring that everything is equally coated.

Spread the wet oat mixture evenly on a large baking sheet covered with parchment paper or lightly coated with oil. Bake 10 to 12 minutes, or until the granola is nicely browned.

Remove from the oven and add the nut and seed mixture, then return to the oven for another 10 to 12 minutes, or until crisp. Remove from the oven and add the dried fruit.

Let cool to room temperature before storing in a glass or plastic airtight jar.

Notes: Made ahead of time, this becomes an easy breakfast on a busy morning. Making your own granola is the best way to control the amount of sugar and fat it contains, as store-bought varieties are often laden with both, in addition to being more expensive.

Rolled oats have been proven to lower cholesterol, enhance immunity, and help to stabilize blood sugar levels (always important in pregnancy). The nuts and seeds provide calcium, protein, essential fats, and other vitamins and minerals. Shredded coconut and ghee increase ojas, and the spices help to lighten and aid in digesting the heaviness of some of the ingredients. You can also use other spices such as cardamom or clove, and add a touch more maple syrup if you like your granola sweeter.

As is, this recipe is best for Kapha and Pitta types. If your Kapha is high, you can use half the amount of nuts. Pitta types can replace the ground ginger with cardamom. Vata types can occasionally enjoy this granola, but to soften it, make sure to heat some milk and soak the granola in it for 5 minutes before eating. My Ayurvedic colleagues may not agree with me on this one, but in warmer weather I love granola with Greek vanilla yogurt, which contains twice the protein of regular yogurt and a good dose of calcium, making it a fantastic, quick pregnancy breakfast. To make it more "Ayurvedic friendly," have your yogurt at room temperature and sprinkle a spice of your choice on top.

For a gluten-free version, buy oats that are labeled "gluten-free," and use rice or garbanzo bean flour instead of wheat or spelt flour.

Lunch and Dinner

BROCCOLI-GINGER AND SOBA STIR-FRY WITH GOMASIO

Serves 4

Ingredients

1 (8-ounce) package of uncooked soba noodles
1 tablespoon extra-virgin olive oil or sunflower oil
1 (1-inch) piece of fresh ginger, peeled and grated
1 pound broccoli
2 tablespoons water
1 ½ cups red pepper, sliced lengthwise in strips
2 tablespoons toasted sesame oil
2 tablespoons soy sauce or tamari
2 tablespoons maple syrup
Gomasio to taste

Directions

Boil water for soba noodles and cook according to package instructions.

Rinse and chop the broccoli into florets. You can peel the tough outer layer of the broccoli stem and cut it into half-inch squares.

Heat olive or sunflower oil in a wok or large skillet. Add ginger and sauté for a few minutes to

Gomasio

Ingredients

2 cups raw, unhulled brown sesame seeds
1 tablespoon sea salt

Directions

Rinse and drain the sesame seeds. Heat them in a large, dry skillet over medium heat, shaking the skillet often, until they are lightly toasted.

When the seeds are fragrant and golden brown, transfer them to a large plate and let them cool. Toast the sea salt for a minute in the same fashion.

Coarsely grind the cooled sesame seeds and sea salt with a mortar and pestle. Transfer to an airtight container. Eat within two weeks for optimum freshness.

infuse the oil. Add the broccoli, stir well, and then add the water. Cover and cook for 4 to 5 minutes, stirring occasionally. Add the red pepper, stir, and cover again.

When the soba noodles are done, drain and rinse them, and return them to the pot. Add toasted sesame oil, soy sauce or tamari, and maple syrup.

Add the noodles to the simmering vegetables and stir well until everything is well blended.

Serve warm in individual bowls and top with gomasio and protein of your choice (see following recipe for Sweet Sesame Baked Tofu, Salmon, or Chicken).

Notes: Soba are Japanese noodles made from buckwheat. These noodles are light yet robust, and contain all eight essential amino acids, including lysine, which is lacking in wheat. Broccoli is packed with vitamins A and C, calcium (great for building your baby's bones), and the always-needed folic acid. Red pepper is a colorful addition and contains vitamins A, C, and B-6.

I love this dish with baked tofu and a sprinkle of gomasio. Gomasio is a condiment made from sesame seeds and sea salt that provides a calcium-rich, hearty topping. You can purchase it in the Asian section of supermarkets or at natural food stores, or make your own.

This dish is relatively tridoshic. Buckwheat is naturally hot and dry, but the rest of the ingredients balance out these qualities, making the dish suitable for all types. Vatas should do fine if their broccoli is well cooked. They can omit the pepper or add carrots in its place. Kapha types can use sunflower oil instead of sesame oil on the noodles, and reduce the amount of tamari (or use a reduced sodium variety) and maple syrup by half. Use brown rice noodles for a gluten-free version.

SWEET SESAME BAKED TOFU, SALMON, OR CHICKEN
Serves 4
Ingredients
1 pound firm organic tofu, wild salmon filet, or organic boneless, skinless chicken
¼ cup tamari or soy sauce
¼ cup apple cider or mirin
2 tablespoons sunflower or extra-virgin olive oil
2 tablespoons maple syrup

1 tablespoon fresh ginger, peeled and grated
1 tablespoon unhulled sesame seeds

Directions
Preheat oven to 375°F.

Slice the tofu horizontally into thirds, and then crosswise to make 12 triangles. Alternatively, slice the salmon or chicken into 4 equal-sized pieces.

Place the tofu, salmon, or chicken in a single layer in a glass baking dish or on a cookie sheet.

Whisk all remaining ingredients together in a bowl. Pour marinade over protein. Sprinkle sesame seeds on top.

Bake tofu for 30 to 40 minutes, or until all marinade has been absorbed and the tofu is nicely browned. Bake salmon or chicken for 20 minutes or until thoroughly cooked to your liking and browned.

Notes: Fresh from the oven, this dish is fantastic served with a whole grain (such as brown rice or quinoa) or added to a noodle dish or soup (such as soba), and topped with freshly sautéed or steamed veggies. You can garnish with fresh cilantro, scallions, and/or gomasio. All the ingredients are readily available at your grocery or natural food store. Mirin is a rice wine used for cooking that can be found in the Asian food section of most supermarkets.

If you are striving for a plant-based diet, eating moderate amounts of tofu can be part of your healthy, whole-foods program. For daily value, ½ cup of tofu gives 10 grams of protein, 25 percent calcium, 11 percent iron, and a good dose of manganese, phosphorous, and selenium. Baking tofu with fresh ginger and tamari, which renders it more suitable for all types, ameliorates its cold, heavy nature.

One-quarter pound of wild salmon delivers about 22 grams of protein and is high in omega-3 fatty acids. The same quantity of white meat chicken has about 35 grams of protein. All body types can enjoy any of these preparations, but Pittas and Kaphas may want to have a smaller portion of salmon due to its oily and fatty nature.

JAZZED-UP QUINOA
Serves 4
Ingredients
1 ½ cups quinoa
3 cups vegetable broth

1 tablespoon extra-virgin olive oil
2 tablespoons lemon juice
1 to 2 tablespoons fresh parsley, chopped
2 tablespoons toasted pine nuts
2 tablespoons currants
Crumbled feta or goat cheese for garnish (optional)

Directions

Rinse the quinoa well. Place quinoa and vegetable broth in a medium-sized pot, and bring to a boil. Lower the heat, cover, and simmer for 20 minutes or until all the broth is absorbed.

Transfer the quinoa to a large bowl. Add the olive oil, lemon juice, parsley, pine nuts, and currants, and mix well.

Garnish with crumbled cheese, if desired.

Notes: I created this dish to jazz up a simple grain and to entice my children. The little bursts of flavor from the pine nuts and currants add an interesting flair. I remember eating quinoa in Bolivia (where it's cultivated) twenty years ago, when it was hardly known in the United States. Now it is much more popular and available in most natural food stores.

Quinoa is referred to as a "super grain" because of its high nutritional profile. Of your daily value, 1 cup cooked has 8 grams of protein, 15 percent iron, 30 percent magnesium, 19 percent folate, and is high in potassium, manganese, phosphorous, and eight essential amino acids. It is gluten free and considered a complete protein.

You can buy packaged vegetable broth or make your own to add more nutrients and savory twists. Pine nuts add a little extra protein, iron, and crunch. Lemon and parsley lighten and refresh. The crumbled cheese gives extra calcium, protein, and a unique flavor combination.

If you want your quinoa jazzier, add more pine nuts, currants, and feta. For a simpler quinoa dish: Rinse 1 cup quinoa well and place in a medium pot with 2 cups water and a pinch of salt. Bring to a boil, reduce the heat, and simmer covered for 15 to 20 minutes. Do not stir while it's cooking or it can become mushy. Cooked just right, it is a fluffy, soft grain. It's yummy topped with sautéed greens and seeds.

I think of quinoa as a tridoshic grain, as it will not aggravate or decrease any dosha strongly, and is easy to digest.

MARGO'S FAVORITE KALE
Serves 2
Ingredients
1 large bunch kale
2 tablespoons extra-virgin olive oil
1 clove garlic, minced
¼ cup water
¼ teaspoon sea salt

Directions
Rinse the kale well. Chop off thick center stem and discard. Slice leaves into 1- to 2-inch wide pieces.

Heat oil in a cast-iron skillet over medium-high heat. When hot, add garlic and stir frequently until fragrant and just slightly golden. Add kale and stir well to ensure it is well coated with the oil and garlic. Add water and cover. Cook for 4 to 5 minutes, stirring occasionally. Add sea salt and mix well.

Eat while it's hot!

Notes: I can never get enough dark leafy greens. I love their taste and nutritional profile. Kale is loaded with essential nutrients, such as calcium, folate, potassium, fiber, and iron; vitamins A (in the form of beta-carotene), C, and K; and provides more nutritional value from fewer calories than almost any other food. It has been shown to have anticancer and immune-boosting properties. Most of all, I love how I feel after I eat it, and really enjoy watching my kids gobble it up.

This recipe is simple, delicious, and can be eaten many times a week, if not daily. You can increase or decrease the olive oil and garlic, according to taste and desire. Garlic adds a pungent flavor and warming energetic with an immune-boosting quality, always beneficial in the colder months. If garlic isn't agreeing with you, substitute with 1 tablespoon of freshly grated ginger and use ghee in place of olive oil.

For a balanced lunch or dinner, eat your greens with a whole grain (such as rice, quinoa, or whole grain pasta) and a protein of your choice. Vata types ought to make sure their greens are well cooked but still gorgeously green, while Pitta and Kapha types can enjoy them lightly cooked. Pitta types can omit the garlic.

RED LENTIL DAL

Serves 8

Ingredients

4 cups red lentils

10 cups water

½ small yellow onion, finely diced

1 to 2 tablespoons ghee or sunflower oil

1 teaspoon cumin seeds

1 teaspoon black mustard seeds

1 pinch hing (asafoetida)

1 clove garlic, minced

1 teaspoon turmeric

1 teaspoon ground coriander

2 teaspoons salt

1 lemon, juiced

1 large handful of fresh cilantro, chopped

Directions

Rinse the lentils, removing any stones. Place lentils and water in a large soup pot and bring to a boil uncovered. Skim off foam, cover, bring the heat to low, and simmer, stirring occasionally, for 30 to 45 minutes, or until done.

While the lentils are cooking, heat the ghee or oil in a small saucepan over medium heat, then add the onion. When the onion becomes translucent, add the cumin seeds, the black mustard seeds, and the hing. When mustard seeds begin to pop, add the garlic and sauté for a couple minutes. Add the turmeric and coriander, and continue to sauté for a few more minutes.

Once the lentils are cooked, add the salt, lemon juice, and the sautéed onion and spice mixture to the soup pot. Bring to a boil to blend, and then turn off the heat.

Add the fresh cilantro.

Serve warm.

Notes: Dal is a stew made from dried lentils, peas, or beans, which are dietary staples in India and its neighboring countries. This is my all-time favorite dal: it's delightful, simple, and quick to make once you get the hang of it. The serving size for this recipe is for eight because my family of four eats it for two dinners, or a dinner and a couple lunches. It's best served with rice or chapattis, a fresh-cooked vegetable, a little yogurt, and some mango or cilantro chutney on the side.

Red lentils are small, salmon-colored beans that can be purchased from a health food store or Indian grocer. Like all lentils, they are nutrient dense, gluten free, low in calories and fat, and low on the glycemic index. One cup delivers 18 grams of protein, so if your bowl has 2 cups in it, that's 36 grams in one meal! Lentils are also high in essential amino acids, iron, fiber, and minerals, which makes them an excellent food in pregnancy.

All spices have special qualities. Most of the ones used here are carminatives (help to dispel gas), digestives (promote digestion), and aid assimilation. Their synergy creates a flavorful yet subtle taste.

This dal is tridoshic, though Pitta types should omit the garlic.

SQUASH, CARROT, AND GINGER SOUP

Serves 6

Ingredients

1 medium to large butternut squash

2 medium sweet potatoes

8 cups water + extra for baking squash

8 medium carrots

3 slices of fresh ginger, ¼-inch thick each

1 (13- or 14-ounce) can of coconut milk

½ tablespoon nutmeg

½ tablespoon coriander

½ tablespoon allspice

2 teaspoons sea salt

Directions

Preheat oven to 375°F.

Cut the squash in half lengthwise. Scoop out the seeds, and place it cut-side down on a baking sheet. Add ¼ inch of water.

Clean and scrub the sweet potatoes, pierce them deeply with a fork, and place on a separate baking sheet.

Bake the squash and the sweet potatoes until soft, about 45 minutes to 1 hour.

While the squash and sweet potatoes are cooking, place 8 cups of water in a large soup pot and begin heating on high.

Scrub the carrots, chop off and discard both ends, and chop into 2-inch pieces.

Add the carrots and ginger to the water and bring it to a boil. Reduce the heat, cover, and simmer for 30 minutes. Turn off the heat and let the carrots and ginger rest in the vegetable broth that's been created.

When the squash and sweet potatoes are baked, remove them from the oven and let them cool. Scoop out the flesh of the squash and add it to the soup pot. Peel the sweet potatoes, cut them into pieces, and add them to the soup.

Add the coconut milk, spices, and salt.

Blend the mixture in a blender or in the pot with a wand mixer until smooth.

Notes: This beautiful orange soup is incredibly nurturing on a cold autumn or winter day. The squash, carrots, and sweet potatoes get their orange color from carotenoids, plant pigments that are converted to vitamin A in the body. These are excellent for the development of your baby's bones, teeth, and eyes. All these veggies also give hearty doses of Vitamin C, folate, and fiber.

I often enjoy this soup topped with lightly roasted pumpkin seeds for a crunchy, nutritious addition. For a well-rounded meal, serve the soup with a whole grain or a slice of warm whole-grain bread, a protein (lentils, tofu, salmon, or chicken), and dark leafy greens.

This soup is perfect as is for Vata types. Pitta types can occasionally eat this when it's prepared as directed, or swap out half of the carrots for another sweet potato. Kapha types can make this soup either with light coconut milk or vegetable broth instead of the regular coconut milk, and replace half of the squash with another four carrots.

Sweets and Baked Goods

SURYA'S THUMBPRINT COOKIES

Makes 24 cookies

Ingredients

1 cup raw almonds

1 cup rolled oats

1 cup whole wheat pastry flour

1 teaspoon cinnamon

1 teaspoon cardamom

½ cup coconut oil, melted (or another light oil)

½ cup maple syrup

Your favorite jam

Directions

Preheat oven to 350°F.

In a blender, separately grind the almonds until you obtain a medium-grain meal, then grind the oats until you obtain a fine meal.

In a large mixing bowl, combine the almonds and oats with the next 5 ingredients.

Form small balls (with about 1 tablespoon of batter) with your hands, and then press your thumb in the center, creating a small indentation. Place the pressed balls on a cookie sheet, and using a teaspoon fill each indentation with jam.

Bake for 10 to 12 minutes.

Notes: These are the healthiest and most delicious cookies I have ever eaten. Many thumbprint cookie recipes are laden with white sugar, white flour, and butter. These are a delightful, wholesome alternative created by my dear friend Surya, a yogini and macrobiotic cook extraordinaire. They quickly become a favorite of anyone who eats just one—if you can limit yourself.

Almonds are chock-full of important minerals: copper, manganese, magnesium, selenium, zinc, potassium, calcium, as well as vitamin E and healthy fats. Grinding the almonds yourself ensures their freshness, although you can purchase almond meal (just ground up almonds) to save time. Rolled oats are full of fiber, B vitamins, iron, and a host of other minerals. Coconut oil adds a rich yet light flavor. If you use another oil, choose something other than olive oil. Cinnamon and cardamom lighten the richness of the maple syrup and oil. Look for a fruit juice-sweetened jam, which tastes the best and has no added sugar. I like raspberry or strawberry. These cookies look beautiful, are wonderful to bring to a pot-luck dinner, and can be enjoyed any time of the year.

Vata and Pitta types can enjoy freely. Kapha types can make their own variety with a smaller amount of sunflower oil instead of the coconut oil, and by increasing the spices by ¼ teaspoon each.

NUTTY PUMPKIN-GINGER MUFFINS

Makes 12 muffins

Ingredients

1 ½ cups unbleached whole wheat flour or white whole wheat flour

½ teaspoon salt

1 cup sucanat, turbinado, or other natural sugar

1 teaspoon baking soda

¼ cup ground flax seeds

1 cup organic pumpkin puree

⅓ cup melted ghee or butter

2 eggs, beaten

¼ cup water

1 teaspoon ground ginger

½ teaspoon nutmeg

1 teaspoon cinnamon

½ teaspoon allspice

1 cup walnuts, toasted and chopped

1 tablespoon crystallized ginger, chopped

Directions

Preheat the oven to 350°F.

Mix the flour, salt, sugar, baking soda, and flax seeds in a large mixing bowl.

In another bowl, combine the pumpkin puree, melted ghee or butter, eggs, water, and the four powdered spices.

Combine the wet and dry ingredients with a few swift strokes. Do not overmix. It's okay for the batter to be a little lumpy.

Fold in the nuts and crystallized ginger.

Spoon the mixture into oiled muffin tins.

Bake for 25 to 30 minutes. The muffins are done when a toothpick stuck in the center of the muffin comes out clean.

Cool muffins on a rack.

Notes: These muffins are a super-easy, healthy treat. Pumpkin provides abundant beta-carotene, walnuts are high in Vitamin E and brain-boosting DHA, and the spices help to lighten and make more digestable the otherwise heavy treat. The puree can also be made from any type of baked winter squash such as butternut or acorn. You can mix everything with a wooden spoon; no electric mixers required. Leave out the walnuts if you don't care for them, or add raisins in their place. Ground flax seeds add a hearty dose of omega-3 fatty acids and fiber.

I loved eating these throughout both of my pregnancies. The extra ginger was perfect for my first trimester queasiness. Although they are best served freshly baked and warm, I used to double the batch and stick a bagful in the freezer to toast for midnight snacks.

These muffins are great for Vata and Pitta types, and okay for Kapha types occasionally. Kapha types can increase the spices by ¼ teaspoon, and use sunflower oil instead of butter.

Enjoy one with a hot cup of tea.

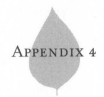

APPENDIX 4

Herbs to Avoid
During Pregnancy

The following herbs are contraindicated during pregnancy; however, some can be used under the guidance of an experienced herbalist. *This is not an exhaustive list.* Used appropriately, many of these herbs can safely be used externally.

Aloe, *Aloe vera*
Angelica, *Angelica archangelica*
Arnica, *Arnica montana*
Ashwagandha, *Withania somnifera*
Barberry, *Berberis vulgaris*
Bee Balm, *Monarda spp.*
Beth root, *Trillium spp.*
Black cohosh (may be used with guidance in the last two weeks of
        pregnancy), *Cimicifuga racemosa*
Black walnut, *Jugulans nigra*
Blessed thistle, *Cnicus benedictus*
Bloodroot, *Sanguinara canadensis*
Blue cohosh (may be used with guidance in the last two weeks of
        pregnancy), *Caulophyllum thalictroides*
Borage, *Borago officinalis*

Buckthorn, *Rhamnus catharticus*
Butternut, *Juglans canadensis*
Calamus, *Acorus calamus*
Calendula, *Calendula officinalis*
Cascara sagrada, *Rhamnus purshiana*
Castor Oil, *Ricinus communis*
Catnip, *Nepeta cataria*
Coltsfoot, *Tussilago farfara*
Comfrey, *Symphytum officinale*
Cotton root, *Gossypum herbaceum*
Damiana, *Turnera aphrodisiaca*
Datura, *Datura spp.*
Dong quai, *Angelica sinensis*
Elecampane, *Inula helenium*
Ephedra, *Ephedra vulgaris*
Fenugreek, *Trigonella foenum-graecum*
Feverfew, *Tanacetum parthenium*
Goldenseal, *Hydrastis canadensis*
Guarana, *Paullinia cupana*
Hops, *Humulus lupulus*
Horehound, *Marrubium vulgare*
Ipecac, *Ipecac ipechachuana*
Jatamansi, *Nardostachys jatamansi*
Juniper berries, *Jupineris spp.*
Kava, *Piper methysticum*
Licorice, *Glycyrrhiza glabra*
Lily of the valley, *Convallaria magalis*
Lobelia, *Lobelia inflata*
Lovage, *Levisticum officinale*
Male fern, *Dryopteris feliz-mas*
Mistletoe, *Viscum album*
Motherwort, *Leonurus cardiaca*
Mugwort, *Artemesia vulgare*
Myrrh, *Commiphora spp.*
Oregon grape root, *Mahonia spp.*
Osha, *Ligusticum porten*
Parsley, *Petroseliunum crispum* (small amounts fine)
Pennyroyal, *Mentha pulegium*

Periwinkle, *Vinca spp.*
Peruvian bark, *Cinchona spp.*
Poke root, *Phytolacca decondra*
Red clover, *Trifolium pratense*
Rhubarb, *Rheum rhabarbarum*
Rue, *Ruta graveolens*
Sage, *Salvia officinalis*
Sarsaparilla, *Smilax officinalis*
Sencio, *Senecio spp.*
Shepherd's purse, *Capsella bursa-pastoris*
Southernwood, *Artemesia absinthium*
Tansy, *Tanacetum vulgare*
Thuja, *Thuja occidentalis*
Uva ursi, *Arctostaphylos uva ursi*
Vitex (can be used the first trimester with guidance), *Vitex angus-castus*
Wormwood, *Artemesia absinthum*
Yarrow, *Achillea millefolium*

APPENDIX 5

How to Make Herbal Oils

Herbal oil is made by infusing or steeping herbs in a nut, seed, or vegetable oil. Making your own is simple and a fun way to enhance the therapeutic benefits of plain oils. Some of my favorite herbs for abhyanga in pregnancy include calendula, renowned for nourishing the skin, and lavender flowers, chamomile flowers, and rose petals, which are all soothing, uplifting, and harmonizing. Sesame, almond, and sunflower oils are most commonly used, but choose the best oil for your dosha (see the table "Dosha-Specific Base Oils"). In Western herbal medicine, olive oil (which is relatively tridoshic, when used externally) is often used in herbal oils. Refer back to the self-massage section in chapter 4 for more information about choosing your oil.

Dosha-Specific Base Oils

AYURVEDIC DOSHA	BEST OILS
Vata	almond, sesame
Pitta	sunflower, coconut
Kapha	sunflower, sesame

Making the Herbal Oil

- Select your herbs and oil.
- Make sure the herbs are clean and dry; if you are using freshly picked flowers, let them sit in the sun for a day to wilt slightly and release excess water stored in them.
- Fill a clean, completely dry quart-sized glass jar with herbs.
- Next, fill the jar to the brim with oil, put the lid on tightly, and shake. You may need to top off the jar with more oil so the herbs are completely covered.
- Place the jar in partial sunlight for one to four weeks. (Many delicate herbs, such as rose petals, require only one week.) Place your jar on an old rag or stone to prevent possible oil stains from seepage. Alternatively, you can pour the contents of the jar into a baking dish and warm it on the lowest setting of your oven (about 120°F to 130°F) for several hours. It is important not to cook or fry the herbs!
- When your time period has finished or after the mixture has cooled, strain the herbs out of the oil using cheesecloth.
- Add a few drops of essential oil (such as lavender or orange) and 400 IU of vitamin E oil.
- Store the oil in a clean, dry bottle and keep it out of direct light and heat. Herbal oil will keep for one year or longer. If it begins to smell rancid (a different odor than the plants you used or the fresh oil), it's no longer good. You can also store your oil in the refrigerator to prolong its shelf life.

How to Use Essential Oils Safely and Effectively

General Guidelines

- Use pure oils, not synthetic fragrances. There is quite a difference in the quality of essential oils available today. See the resources section for reputable companies that sell pure, high-quality essential oils.
- Do not take essential oils internally or apply them directly to the skin without the guidance of a skilled practitioner.
- Keep oils from coming into direct contact with mucus membranes or the eyes.
- Keep oils out of reach of children.
- Citrus oils, such as bergamot, should be used in low dilutions, and you should always avoid contact with UV rays after applying them to the skin.
- Avoid prolonged exposure to essential oils if you're not in a room or area with proper ventilation.
- Store essential oils in a cool environment to avoid rancidity.

How to Use Essential Oils

Baths. Add 5 to 10 drops of oils after the water is drawn and disperse them before getting in the tub. You can also add oils to salts such as Epsom or Dead Sea salts (5 to 10 drops of oil for ½ to 1 cup of salt), mix, and then add to bath water. Use mild, nonirritating oils, such as lavender.

Massage. Always dilute essential oils in carrier oils (nut, seed, or fruit oils, such as almond, sesame, or coconut) for massage. Use about 15 drops of an essential oil for a 1-ounce bottle of massage oil. For children under twelve years of age, use about 6 drops per 1-ounce bottle of massage oil.

Atomizer. An atomizer is a spray device used to disperse an oil, or more commonly, a blend of oils, into the air, onto an object, or onto the body. Add 10 to 50 drops of essential oil (single oil or combination of oils) to a 4-ounce bottle of pure water.

Facial steam. Add 1 to 4 drops of essential oil to a pot of boiling water (about 4 cups). Place your head over the pot and cover the pot and head with a towel. Stay for about 5 minutes.

Compress. Add 10 drops essential oil to a basin of hot water (about 4 ounces). Soak a washcloth, wring it out, and apply to desired area.

Direct palm inhalation. This method is useful for oils that can safely be applied to the skin (such as lavender or sandalwood). Apply 1 to 2 drops of oil on palms, rub hands together, and inhale.

Diffusers. There are many types of diffusers available today. Follow the instructions that come with your diffuser to determine the number of drops to use.

Essential Oils That Can Be Used in Pregnancy

In a normal, healthy pregnancy, the following oils can be used carefully after the first trimester. (This is not an exhaustive list.)

Bergamot
Chamomile
Cypress
Eucalyptus
Frankincense
Geranium
Ginger
Grapefruit
Lavender
Neroli
Rose
Rosewood
Sandalwood
Sweet orange
Tangerine
Tea tree
Ylang ylang

ACKNOWLEDGMENTS

To my teachers of Ayurveda: Dr. David Frawley, Dr. Vasant Lad, and Bri Maya Tiwari. Your influence on my life and work is immeasurable.

To my teachers of yoga, especially Sonia Nelson and T. K. V. Desikachar. Thank you, Sonia, for being an extraordinary mentor and for guiding me carefully through the creation of this book.

Eternal gratitude to Nicolai, my beloved husband, for his unwavering support and encouragement, and incredible partnership. Thank you for helping me fulfill my *dharma* in completing this book. Your high-*Pitta* editing skills have been exceptional! Your devotion to our family is a true blessing. I love you.

I am grateful to everyone at Sounds True (especially Haven Iverson, Jennifer Brown, Amy Rost, and Tami Simon) for believing in this book, trusting me to write it, and taking a step out of your normal publishing goals to see it manifest. It has been a delight to work with such a spirited and dedicated team.

To my parents, Pat and Dick Shapiro. Mom, I am fortunate to have you as my first teacher, writing coach, and dearest friend. Thank you for your steadfast support and encouragement all the way through and for the endless hours babysitting your grandchildren! Dad, thank you for always encouraging me to educate myself, believing in me, and being a continuous loving presence in my life.

To all the readers and editors of the many versions of this book: Nicolai Bachman, Pat Shapiro, Sonia Nelson, Sandra Ortsman, Patricia Rosen CNM, FNP, Dr. Sharada Hall, and Dr. Diane Friedman, MD. And especially Jade Groff CNM, soul sister, colleague, and beloved friend for so many years—thank you for your insights, editing, being my sounding board, and awesome support.

To my students and clients for allowing me to be your guide.

To my girlfriends, near and far, who have deeply supported me on this journey. Thank you for being part of my life.

To the plants and Mother Earth for letting me work with your gifts.

Finally, to my children, Sierra and Mateo, for giving me the opportunity to become a mother and try, firsthand, almost everything in this book. Your lives are the greatest gifts to me. You bless me each and every day. Thank you for your patience while I birthed my "third child."

Resources

AUTHOR

Margo Bachman, MA, RYT500
The Heart of Wellness
PO Box 4352
Santa Fe, NM 87502
margoshapirobachman.com

   Margo offers consultations in person, by phone, or video, as well as workshops on Ayurveda, yoga, and herbal medicine, specializing in women's and children's health.

Ayurveda

BULK HERBS, FORMULAS, AND AYURVEDIC HEALTH SUPPLIES

Banyan Botanicals, banyanbotanicals.com
The Ayurvedic Institute, shop.ayurveda.com

JOURNALS

Light on Ayurveda: Journal of Health, loaj.com/ayurvedic_journal.html
Ayurveda Today, quarterly journal of the Ayurvedic Institute, see shop.ayurveda.com

POSTPARTUM CARE

Sacred Window School for Maternal and Newborn Health (sacredwindow.com) offers trainings and resources in Ayurvedic postpartum care.

PRACTITIONERS

The National Ayurvedic Medical Association (NAMA, ayurvedanama.org) is the only governing body of Ayurvedic practitioners in the

United States. See its online practitioner directory, under Find a Professional, to find a qualified practitioner near you.

SCHOOLS IN THE UNITED STATES

American Institute of Vedic Studies (based in Santa Fe, NM, but distance learning), vedanet.com

The Ayurvedic Institute (Albuquerque, NM), ayurveda.com

California College of Ayurveda (Nevada City, CA), ayurvedacollege.com

Kripalu School of Ayurveda (Lenox, MA), kripalu.org/study_with_us/351

Mount Madonna College of Ayurveda (Watsonville, CA), mountmadonnainstitute.org/ayurveda

Essential Oils

DōTerra, doterra.com

Floracopeia, floracopeia.com

Mountain Rose Herbs, mountainroseherbs.com

HERBS, HERBAL SUPPLIES, AND OTHER SUPPLEMENTS

Avena Botanicals, avenabotanicals.com, is a small company with wonderful handcrafted herbal products.

Frontier Coop, frontiercoop.com, offers bulk organic herbs, spices, and teas.

Motherlove, motherlove.com, offers herbal products for pregnancy, birth, breastfeeding, and babies.

Mountain Rose Herbs, mountainroseherbs.com, carries an extensive selection of bulk herbs, spices, essential oils, and other cool stuff.

New Chapter Prenatal Vitamins, newchapter.com/prenatal, are based on whole foods for healthy pregnancy and fetal development.

Nordic Naturals, nordicnaturals.com, carries Prenatal DHA and Algae Omega (vegetarian DHA).

HERBAL ORGANIZATIONS

American Botanical Council, abc.herbalgram.org

The American Herbalists Guild, americanherbalistsguild.com

ORGANIC PRODUCE

The Environmental Working Group analyzes the Department of Agriculture's data about pesticide residue and ranks foods based on how much or little pesticide residue they have. Its "Dirty Dozen" and "Clean Fifteen" are annually updated lists of produce with the highest and lowest pesticide residues, respectively. For the most current lists, see ewg.org/foodnews.

PREGNANCY, BIRTH, AND BREASTFEEDING

American College of Nurse-Midwives, midwife.org
Birthing From Within, birthingfromwithin.com
Doulas of North America (DONA) International, dona.org
La Leche League International, llli.org
Midwives Alliance of North America, mana.org
Mothering, an online community and magazine for natural family living, mothering.com

VEDIC CHANT

The Vedic Chant Center (Sonia Nelson, director; vedicchantcenter.org) offers classes, workshops, and CDs.

YOGA MATS AND OTHER SUPPLIES

Hugger Mugger, huggermugger.com
Jade Yoga Mats, jadeyoga.com
Manduka, manduka.com/us

YOGA TEACHER

Healing Yoga Foundation (healingyoga.org) offers teacher training programs and a resource directory of teachers trained in the tradition of T. Krishnamacharya and T. K. V. Desikachar.

RECOMMENDED READING

Ayurveda and Yoga

Bachman, Nicolai. *The Language of Yoga*. Boulder, Colorado: Sounds True, 2005.
Desikachar, T. K. V. *The Heart of Yoga: Developing a Personal Practice*. Rochester, Vermont: Inner Traditions International, 1995.
Frawley, Dr. David. *Ayurvedic Healing*. Twin Lakes, Wisconsin: Lotus Press, 2000.

Frawley, Dr. David and Lad, Dr. Vasant. *The Yoga of Herbs*. Twin Lakes, Wisconsin: Lotus Press, 1988.

Kraftsow, Gary. *Yoga for Wellness: Healing with the Timeless Teachings of Viniyoga*. New York, New York: Penguin Group, 1999.

Lad, Vasant. *Ayurveda: The Science of Self-Healing*. Santa Fe, New Mexico: Lotus Press, 1984.

Svoboda, Robert E. *Prakriti: Your Ayurvedic Constitution*. Twin Lakes, Wisconsin: Lotus Press, 1998.

Women's Health and Pregnancy

England, Pam and Horowitz, Rob. *Birthing From Within*. Albuquerque, New Mexico: Partera Press, 1998.

Gaskin, Ina May. *Ina May's Guide to Childbirth*. New York, New York: Bantam Books, 2003.

Northrup, Christine. *Women's Bodies, Women's Wisdom*. New York, New York: Bantam Books, 2002.

Parvati, Jeannine. *Hygieia, A Woman's Herbal*. Freestone Press, 1992.

Romm, Aviva Jill. *The Natural Pregnancy: Herbs, Nutrition, and Other Holistic Choices*. Berkeley, California: Celestial Arts, 2003.

Romm, Aviva. *Botanical Medicine for Women's Health*. St. Louis, Missouri: Churchill Livingstone, 2010.

Svoboda, Robert E. *Ayurveda for Women*. Rochester, Vermont: Healing Arts Press, 2000.

Tiwari, Bri Maya. *The Path of Practice: A Woman's Book of Healing with Food, Breath, and Sound*. New York: Ballantine Books, 2000.

Welch, Claudia. *Balance Your Hormones, Balance Your Life; Achieving Optimal Health and Wellness through Ayurveda, Chinese Medicine, and Western Science*. Cambridge, Massachusetts: De Capo Press, 2011.

COOKBOOKS AND RECIPES

Katzen, Mollie. *The New Moosewood Cookbook*. Berkeley, California: Ten Speed Press, 2000.

McEachern, Leslie. *The Angelica Home Kitchen: Recipes and Rabble Rousings from an Organic Vegan Restaurant*. Berkeley, California: Ten Speed Press, 2003.

Morningstar, Amadea, with Urmila Desai. *The Ayurvedic Cookbook*. Santa Fe, New Mexico: Lotus Press, 1990.

Somerville, Annie. *Field of Greens: New Vegetarian Recipes from the Celebrated Greens Restaurant*. New York, New York: Bantam Books, 1993.

Tiwari, Bri Maya. *Ayurveda: A Life of Balance*. Rochester, Vermont: Healing Arts Press, 1995.

Check out recipes on my website: margoshapirobachman.com

GLOSSARY

Quotation marks indicate the direct English translation of the Sanskrit.

Abhyanga. Full-body oil massage.

Agni. "Fire," digestive/metabolic fire.

Anabolic. A force in the body that causes growth and development.

Angula. "Finger unit" used for measuring **marma points.**

Apana vayu. "Downward air."

Asafoetida. A spice also known as hing, used in very small amounts in Indian cooking.

Asana. "Seat, sitting," referring to a yoga posture.

Bhavana. Idea, attitude, or intention.

Breech. Refers to a baby whose buttocks or feet are presented first at the end of pregnancy and during the birth process.

Buddhi. The individual intellect.

Chyavanprash. A rejuvenating herbal jam made primarily from amalaki fruit with other herbs, spices, sugar, and ghee.

Complete. Refers to a woman fully dilated in labor.

Contraction. The shortening and thickening of a muscle.

Dauhrdini. "Two hearted," referring to a pregnant woman.

Dharana. "Keeping the attention on a single place."

Dharma. Duty, law, or personal path.

Dhatu. Structural tissues that make up the human body.

Dhyana. Continuous focus.

Dilation. The opening of the cervix in labor.

Dinacharya. Daily routine.

Dosha. "Defect," bodily humor/force, fault, imperfection.

Doula. A woman who provides continuous physical, emotional, and informational support before, during, and just after birth, and/or during postpartum.

Epidural. A local anesthetic that is administered into a spinal space in the lower back.

Episiotomy. An incision made into the perineum and vagina to surgically widen the birth passage.

Fontanels. Soft spots on a baby's head which, during birth, enable the bony plates of the skull to flex, allowing the child's head to pass through the birth canal.

Ghee. Clarified butter.

Guna. Attribute or quality.

Infusion. A medicinal-strength tea made from steeping herbs in water.

Ishvara pranidhana. An attitude of not being attached to the fruits of your actions.

Kapha. One of the three biological humors comprised of the earth and water elements.

Karma. Action; also refers to a principle in which every action creates an opposite reaction.

Mantra. Sound that yields an energetic effect.

Marma point. "Vulnerable" or "sensitive" area; pressure points throughout the body where **prana** is concentrated.

Meconium. The first fecal excretion of a newborn child.

Nadi. "River," channel or passageway.

Neti pot. A small ceramic pot filled with warm salt water to rinse and cleanse the sinuses.

Ojas. Strength of the immune system and a subtle essence of **Kapha dosha.**

Panchakarma. "Five actions," Ayurvedic cleansing treatments.

Pitocin. A synthetic hormone given intravenously to induce or accelerate labor.

Pitta. One of the three biological humors comprised of the fire and water elements.

Placenta. The blood-rich organ attached to the inside wall of the uterus that nourishes the baby during pregnancy.

Prakruti. One's biological constitution from birth and referring to the fundamental principle of matter.

Prana. The vital life force, breath, and a subtle essence of **Vata dosha.**

Pranayama. Control or regulation of **prana** to improve the quality of awareness and perception.

Progesterone. A naturally occurring hormone in the female reproductive system that supports pregnancy.

Purusha. The fundamental principle of one's spirit or infinite consciousness.

Rajas. One of the three universal qualities or **gunas** of movement, activity, and energy.

Rasayana. A rejuvenating substance.

Samadhi. A balanced state of body, mind, and consciousness.

Sattva. One of the three universal qualities or **gunas** of clarity, consciousness, intelligence, and balance.

Shakti. Power, ability, energy.

Snehana. "Love," the process of internal and external oil applications.

Subdosha. Five subsets of the doshas that perform different functions.

Svadhyaya. Self-observation.

Tamas. One of the three universal qualities or **gunas** of inertia, darkness, and heaviness.

Tejas. Brilliance or fire of the immune system and a subtle essence of **Pitta dosha.**

Trataka. "To look" or "gaze," a traditional meditation practice in which you gaze at a candle flame.

Tridoshic. Referring to something that is good for all doshic types.

Upanishads. Texts compiled after the Vedas (spiritual literature from ancient Indian culture).

Vata. One of the three biological humors comprised of the air and ether elements.

Vena Cava. Either of two large veins returning blood into the right atrium of the heart.

Vikruti. Current, imbalanced state of an individual.

Yogini. A woman who practices yoga.

Yoni. Vagina.

BIBLIOGRAPHY

BOOKS AND JOURNAL ARTICLES

Albers, L. L., et al. "Midwifery Care Measures in the Second Stage of Labor and Reduction of Genital Tract Trauma at Birth: a Randomized Trial." *Journal of Midwifery & Women's Health* (2005), 365–372.

Athavale, V. B. *Bala Veda, Pediatrics and Ayurveda*. Delhi: Chaukhamba Sanskrit Pratishthan, 2000.

Bachman, Margo. "Insights on Pregnancy from Yoga and Ayurveda." *Yoga Therapy Today* (March 2010), 12–14.

Bachman, Nicolai. *The Language of Ayurveda*. Victoria: Trafford Publishing, 2005.

Campbell, Andrew W. "Organic vs. Conventional." *Alternative Therapies* 18, no. 6 (Nov/Dec 2012), 8–9.

Coletta, Jaclyn, MD, et al. "Omega-3 Fatty Acids and Pregnancy," *Reviews in Obstetrics and Gynecology*. (Fall 2010); 3(4), 163–171.

Crow, David. *The Pharmacy of Flowers*. Nevada City: Floracopeia, 2005.

Deardorff, Julie. "Risk of Disease Linked to Fetal Life; Study Finds Certain Illnesses Can be Rooted to Time Spent in Womb." *Chicago Tribune*. Accessed in *SF New Mexican*, November 26, 2011.

de Boer, Hugo, and Vichith Lamxay. "Plants used during pregnancy, childbirth and postpartum healthcare in Lao PDR: A comparative study of the Brou, Saek and Kry ethnic groups." *Journal of Ethnobiology and Ethnomedicine* (2009), 5:25.

Desikachar, T. K. V. *The Heart of Yoga: Developing a Personal Practice*. Rochester, Vermont: Inner Traditions International, 1995.

Desikachar, T. K. V., et al. *The Viniyoga of Yoga: Applying Yoga for Healthy Living*. Chennai: Krishnamacharya Yoga Mandiram, 2001.

England, Pam, and Rob Horowitz. *Birthing From Within*. Albuquerque, New Mexico: Partera Press, 1998.

Field, T., et al. "Massage Therapy for Infants of Depressed Mothers." *Infant Behavior and Development*, (1996); 19, 107–112.

Field, T., et al. "Pregnant Women Benefit from Massage Therapy." *J Psychosom. Obstet. Gynaecol.* (Mar 1999); 20(1): 31–8.

Frawley, David. *Ayurvedic Healing: A Comprehensive Guide*. Twin Lakes: Lotus Press, 2000.

Frawley, D., and S. Kozak. *Yoga for Your Type*. Twin Lakes: Lotus Press, 2001.

Gaskin, Ina May. *Ina May's Guide to Childbirth*. New York, New York: Bantam Books, 2003.

Goyal, R. K., J. Singh, and H. Lal. "*Asparagus racemosus*—an update." *Indian J Med Sci* (2003); 57:408.

Joshi, Nirmala G. *Ayurvedic Concepts in Gynecology*. Delhi: Chaukhamba Sanskrit Pratishthan, 1999.

Kraftsow, Gary. *Yoga for Wellness: Healing with the Timeless Teachings of Viniyoga*. New York: Penguin Group, 1999.

Krishnamacharya, T. *Sri Nathamuni's Yogarahasya*. Chennai: Krishnamacharya Yoga Mandiram, 1988.

Kumaramangalam, Bharati. *Textbook of Prasuti Tantra*. Varanasi: Chowkhamba Krishnadas Academy, 2008.

Labrecque, Michel, et al. "Randomized controlled trial of prevention of perineal trauma by perineal massage during pregnancy." *American Journal of Obstetrics & Gynecology* 180 (March 1999); Issue 3, 593–600.

Lad, Vasant. *Pregnancy and Infant Care Audio Tape*. Albuquerque: The Ayurvedic Institute, 1998.

———. *Textbook of Ayurveda: Complete Guide to Clinical Assessment*. Albuquerque: The Ayurvedic Institute, 2006.

———. *Textbook of Ayurveda: Fundamental Principles*. Albuquerque: The Ayurvedic Institute, 2002.

Lad, Vasant, and Anisha Durve. *Marma Points of Ayurveda*. Albuquerque: The Ayurvedic Institute, 2008.

Levy, Juliette de Bairacli. *Nature's Children*. Woodstock: Ash Tree Publishing, 1997.

Lim, Robin. *After the Baby's Birth . . . A Woman's Way to Wellness: A Complete Guide for Postpartum Women*. Berkeley, California: Celestial Arts, 1991.

Low Dog, Tieraona. "The Use of Botanicals During Pregnancy and Lactation." *Alternative Therapies* 15, no. 1 (Jan/Feb 2009), 54–58.

Morningstar, Amadea, with Urmila Desai. *The Ayurvedic Cookbook*. Santa Fe, New Mexico: Lotus Press, 1990.

Murthy, K. R., Srikantha, trans. *Ashtanga Hrdayam, Volume 1*. Varanasi: Krishnadas Academy, 1991.

"Noise: a Hazard for the Fetus and Newborn," *American Academy of Pediatrics*. Committee on Environmental Health (Oct 1997): 724–7.

Oaks, Ysha. *Touching Heaven; Tonic Postpartum Care from Ayurveda*. Self-published by SWA MA CHI, 2003.

Pole, Sebastian. *Ayurvedic Medicine: The Principles of Traditional Practice*. Philadelphia: Elsevier, 2006.

———. *Botanical Medicine for Women's Health*. St. Louis, MO: Churchill Livingstone, 2010.

———. "Herbs for the Mom-to-Be; Sound advice for using medicinal plants to treat common pregnancy ailments." *Mothering Magazine* (2008), 54–61.

Romm, Aviva Jill. *The Natural Pregnancy: Herbs, Nutrition and Other Holistic Choices*. Berkeley: Celestial Arts, 2003.

Roseboom, Tessa J., et al. "Effects of Prenatal Exposure to the Dutch Famine on Adult Disease in Later Life: An Overview." *Molecular and Cellular Endocrinology*, 185 (2001), 93–98.

Sachs, Melanie. *Ayurvedic Beauty Care: Ageless Techniques to Invoke Natural Beauty*. Delhi: Motilal Banarsidass, 1998.

Sharma, Priyavrat, editor and trans. *Charaka Samhita* 1. Delhi: Chaukhamba Orientalia, 1981.

Sharma, Priya Vrat, editor and trans. *Sushruta-Samhita* 2. Varanasi: Chaukhamba Visvabharti, 2000.

Spackman, Linda, and Prajna Yoga. *Yoga & Pregnancy: An In-Depth Study*. Santa Fe: Prajna Yoga, 2010.

Svoboda, Robert E. *Ayurveda for Women: A Guide to Vitality and Health*. Rochester, VT: Healing Arts Press, 2000.

Tewari, Premvati. *Ayurvediya Prasuti-Tantra Evam Stri-Roga*, Parts 1 and 2. Varanasi: Chaukhambha Orientalia, 2009.

Tiwari, Bri Maya. *Ayurveda: A Life of Balance*. Rochester, VT: Healing Arts Press, 1995.

Willetts, K., et al. "Effect of a ginger extract on pregnancy-induced nausea: A randomized controlled trial." *Aust N Z J Obstet Gynaecol*. (2003); 43(2): 139–144.

ONLINE SOURCES

"About Pulses: Health and Nutrition," webpage on the USA Dry Pea and Lentil Council website (no date), cookingwithpulses.com/about-pulses/health-nutrition/. Accessed April 3, 2013.

"Best Foods to Eat While Pregnant," article on the website *What to Expect* (no date). Available at whattoexpect.com/pregnancy/eating-well/week-11/big-nutrition-small-packages.aspx. Accessed April 3, 2013.

"Counseling Postpartum Patients About Diet and Exercise," clinical fact sheet on the Association for Reproductive Health Professionals website (July 2008). Available at arhp.org/publications-and-resources/clinical-fact-sheets/postpartum-counseling.

"Healing Foods: Fruit and Veggies Recipes: Blueberries," *Vegetarian Times*, article online (no date). Available at vegetariantimes.com/article/blue-berries2/. Accessed April 3, 2013.

"Healing Foods: Grains & Legumes Recipes: Quinoa," *Vegetarian Times*, article online (no date). Available at vegetariantimes.com/article/heal-ing-foods-quinoa/. Accessed April 3, 2013.

"Nutrients and Vitamins for Pregnancy," article on the American Pregnancy Association website (January 2013). Available at americanpregnancy.org/pregnancyhealth/nutrientsvitaminspregnancy.html.

"Pregnancy and Headaches," article on the American Pregnancy Association website (March 2007). Available at americanpregnancy.org/pregnancyhealth/headaches.html.

"Protein: Moving Closer to Center Stage," article on the Harvard School for Public Health website (no date). Available at hsph.harvard.edu/nutritionsource/protein-full-story/. Accessed April 4, 2013.

"Why Use a Doula?" webpage on the DONA International website (no date). Available at dona.org/mothers/why_use_a_doula.php. Accessed April 3, 2013.

Ehrlich, Steven D. "Omega 3 Fatty Acids," article on the University of Maryland Medical Center website (May 10, 2011). Available at umm.edu/altmed/articles/omega-3-000316.htm#ixzz1mCdW3f2s.

Food and Nutrition Board, Institute of Medicine (IOM) of the National Academies. "Table: Recommended Dietary Allowance and Adequate Intake Values, Vitamins and Elements," from "Dietary Reference Intakes Tables and Application," background information on the "Summary Report of the Dietary Reference Intakes" (September 15, 2006). Available for download at iom.edu/Activities/Nutrition/SummaryDRIs/DRI-Tables.aspx.

Krucoff, Carol. "Positively Healing," article on the *Yoga Journal* website. Available at yogajournal.com/practice/2570. Accessed June 3, 2012.

Lack, Evonne. "The Best Ten Foods for Pregnancy," article on the website BabyCenter (no date). Available at babycenter.com/0_the-ten-best-foods-for-pregnancy_10320506.bc. Accessed April 3, 2013.

Mayo Clinic staff. "Pregnancy Week by Week," article on the Mayo Clinic website (March 19, 2011). Available at mayoclinic.com/health/pregnancy-week-by-week/MY00331.

Mayo Clinic staff. "Pregnancy Week by Week: Fetal Development: The First Trimester," article on the Mayo Clinic website (December 4, 2012). Available at mayoclinic.com/health/prenatal-care/PR00112.

Mayo Clinic staff. "Pregnancy Week by Week: Prenatal Yoga: What You Need to Know," article on the Mayo Clinic website (January 22, 2013). Available at mayoclinic.com/health/prenatal-yoga/MY01542.

Pau, Jackie. "The Dirty Dozen and Clean 15 of Produce," article on the PBS website (May 13, 2010). Available at pbs.org/wnet/need-to-know/health/the-dirty-dozen-and-clean-15-of-produce/616/.

World Health Organization. "Health Topics: Breastfeeding," undated webpage. Available at who.int/topics/breastfeeding/en/. Accessed April 3, 2013.

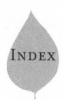

INDEX

Page numbers in italics indicate figures or tables.

About the Author

Margo Shapiro Bachman, MA, RYT500, is a nationally certified Ayurvedic practitioner with an MA in education and a BS in botanical science. She has spent over twenty years immersed in the study and practice of Western herbal medicine. Margo's Ayurvedic training has been primarily through private and small group study with Dr. David Frawley, Dr. Vasant Lad, and Bri Maya Tiwari. Margo has been a private student of Dr. Frawley's for over ten years. She received additional clinical training from Dr. Lad at The Ayurvedic Institute. A yoga and meditation practitioner for over twenty years, she teaches prenatal yoga and therapeutic applications of yoga. She studied at the Krishnamacharya Yoga Mandiram, one of the leading educational institutions for yoga therapy in India, and continues to study yoga therapy, yoga philosophy, and Vedic chanting with Sonia Nelson in New Mexico. Margo loves making the ancient teachings of Ayurveda and yoga accessible, understandable, and relevant to modern life. Her private practice and teaching focus on women's and children's health. Margo lives in Santa Fe, New Mexico with her husband and two children. For more information, please visit her website, margoshapirobachman.com

ABOUT SOUNDS TRUE

Sounds True is a multimedia publisher whose mission is to inspire and support personal transformation and spiritual awakening. Founded in 1985 and located in Boulder, Colorado, we work with many of the leading spiritual teachers, thinkers, healers, and visionary artists of our time. We strive with every title to preserve the essential "living wisdom" of the author or artist. It is our goal to create products that not only provide information to a reader or listener, but that also embody the quality of a wisdom transmission.

For those seeking genuine transformation, Sounds True is your trusted partner. At SoundsTrue.com you will find a wealth of free resources to support your journey, including exclusive weekly audio interviews, free downloads, interactive learning tools, and other special savings on all our titles.

To learn more, visit SoundsTrue.com/bonus/free-gifts or call us toll free at 800-333-9185.

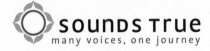